Essentials of
Veterinary Toxicology

The Editor

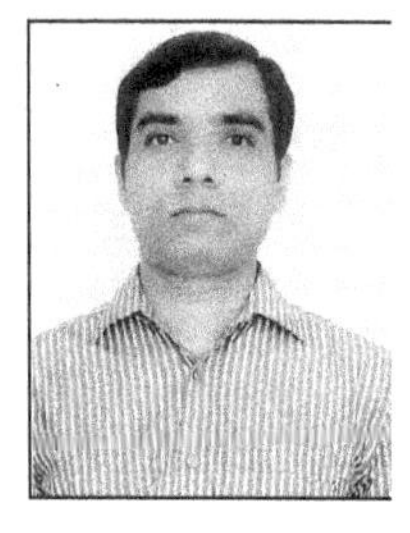

Naveen Kumar obtained graduation (B.V.Sc. and A.H.) from College of Veterinary Science and Animal Husbandry, Bhubaneswar, OUAT, Orissa and master's (M.V.Sc.) with academic distinction in Veterinary Pharmacology and Toxicology from Ranchi Veterinary College, BAU, Jharkhand. He started early career as a Teaching Personnel in Department of Veterinary Clinics, College of Veterinary and Animal Sciences, GBPUA&T, Pantnagar; then joined Khalsa College of Veterinary and Animal Sciences (KCVAS), Amritsar as an Assistant Professor in the Department of Veterinary Pharmacology and Toxicology. He has published several research and popular articles in different journals. He has qualified ICAR-SRF (PGS) examination in the discipline of Veterinary Pharmacology. Later he was selected for Senior Research Fellowship (SRF) by University Grants Commission (UGC), New Delhi and currently pursuing Ph.D. in the Department of Veterinary Pharmacology and Toxicology, College of Veterinary and Animal Sciences, GBPUA&T, Pantnagar.

He is a life member of professional societies including, Veterinary Council of India (VCI); Indian Society of Veterinary Pharmacology and Toxicology (ISVPT); Society of Toxicology (STOX), India and Indian Pharmacology Society (IPS).

Essentials of
Veterinary Toxicology

— Editor —

Naveen Kumar

2019

Daya Publishing House®

A Division of

Astral International Pvt. Ltd.
New Delhi – 110 002

© 2019 EDITOR

ISBN: 9789389569056 (Int. Edition)

Published by : **Daya Publishing House®**
A Division of
Astral International Pvt. Ltd.
– ISO 9001:2015 Certified Company –
4736/23, Ansari Road, Darya Ganj
New Delhi-110 002
Ph. 011-43549197, 23278134
E-mail: info@astralint.com
Website: www.astralint.com

Digitally Printed at : **Replika Press Pvt. Ltd.**

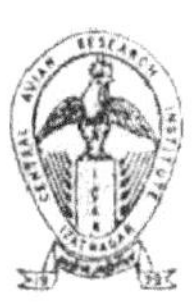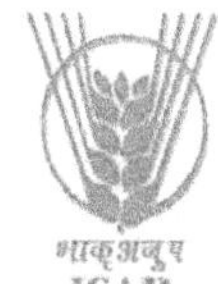

Foreword

It gives me immense pleasure to recommend this textbook titled *"Essentials of Veterinary Toxicology"* edited by Dr. Naveen Kumar which is being published for use-by thousands of undergraduate students of veterinary sciences. It is always welcome to author a textbook that specially addresses the needs of young U.G students and simultaneously help-arouse a passion for pharmacology in particular, for pursuing it through specialization. I am glad that these basic purposes have been given due care by the authors.

The material included chapters of this book covers all major syllabus of veterinary toxicology laid down by Veterinary Council of India (VCI) which are mandatory and covered in all veterinary colleges. It is then a privilege to offer most required facets through this textbook. If I recollect, there are only few books available in markets which satisfy all basic requirements of students. Thus, the present book "Essentials of Veterinary Toxicology" will fulfill the need of graduate students and U.G teachers as well. I find most chapters adequately cover the important needs of veterinary pharmacology and toxicology, a knowledge-sphere of a veterinary student which should precede his practice of veterinary medicines, through the final years of BVSc curriculum.

The other important aim of the book is to help students in coping with problems arising 'from various competitive exams. Every attempt is visibly made here to make the book easily readable and understandable by students who come from a wide spectrum of educational backgrounds. New concept is introduced to summarize the essential points. In addition, this book also brings insight for future veterinarians on the newest approaches for diagnosing poisoning cases in all animals from chemicals and plants of a diverse nature. Hope this textbook help to students with a clear basic idea and concepts of what students are expected to do better. May this book provide effective stimulus for the students to gain knowledge and endure a successful journey of Veterinary practitioner armed with latest inputs of Toxicology. Lastly, I admire the author and publishers for the accomplishment in cataloguing yet another veterinary pharmacology text book in history of Veterinary Education of the country.

Dhirendra Kumar

Ph.D.

Scientist

Preface

The material included within the chapter of this book covers all the syllabus of veterinary toxicology laid down by the Veterinary Council of India (VCI), New Delhi India that are mandatory and followed by all veterinary colleges. It is our privilege to share some facets through this book. I wish to thanks all the contributors for making it happen. There are only few books available in markets which satisfy all the basic and competitive requirement of students. This book could serve the basic knowledge of toxicology field. Present book **"Essentials of Veterinary Toxicology"** will fulfill the needs of graduate students. The cooperation, suggestion and encouragement by our family members, teachers, seniors and friends for their continuing availability in time of need are highly appreciable.

The main aim of the book is to help the students in coping with the problems arising from various competitive exams. Every attempt has been made to make the book easily readable and understandable by students who come from a wide spectrum of educational backgrounds. New concept is introduced to summarize the essential points. Hope this textbook help to students with a clear basic idea and concept of what students are expected. May this book provide effective stimulus for the students to gain knowledge and ease their journey through a fascinating materials with latest information. Although effort has been carried out to maintain the accuracy of information contained in this edition, neither the Editor nor its Author assumes any responsibility for consequences which may arise from its use.

I humbly welcome the valuable suggestions and constructive criticism from the readers for further improvement of this book in subsequent editions. I express my sincere gratitude and congratulations to all authors for their unstinted support. I am thankful to Publisher, Astral International Pvt. Ltd., New Delhi, India for his dedicated support.

Naveen Kumar

Contents

List of Contributors

Dr. Rajeev Ranjan, *M.V.Sc., Ph.D.*

Assistant Professor,

Veterinary Pharmacology and Toxicology,

College of Veterinary Science and Animal Husbandry

Rewa – 486 001, Madhya Pradesh

Dr. C. V. Savalia, *M.V.Sc., Ph.D.*

Professor and Head

Veterinary Public Health and Epidemiology,

College of Veterinary Science and Animal Husbandry

NAU, Navsari – 396 450, Gujarat

Dr. Amita Ranjan, *M.V.Sc., Ph.D.*

Assistant Professor,

Department of Veterinary Pharmacology and Toxicology,

College of Veterinary and Animal Sciences (RAJUVAS),

Bikaner - 334001, Rajasthan

Dr. Rajeev Kumar, *M.V.Sc., Ph.D.*

Assistant Professor,

Veterinary Public Health and Epidemiology,

College of Veterinary Science and Animal Husbandry

NAU, Navsari – 396 450, Gujarat

Dr. Disha Pant, *M.V.Sc.*

Assistant Professor

Veterinary Pharmacology and Toxicology,

CVASc, GBPUAT,

Pantnagar – 263 145, Uttarakhand

Dr. Rakesh Ranjan, *M.V.Sc., Ph.D.*

Senior Scientist,

ICAR-National Research Centre on Camel, Bikaner - 334001, Rajasthan

Dr. Jeevan Ranjan Dash, *M.V.Sc., Ph.D.*
Assistant Professor
Pharmacology and Toxicology,
College of Veterinary Science,
OUAT, Bhubaneswar – 751 003, Odisha

Dr. Ratn Deep Singh, *M.V.Sc., Ph.D.*
Assistant Professor
Veterinary Pharmacology and Toxicology,
College of Veterinary Science and Animal Husbandry
SDAU, S.K. Nagar – 385 506, Gujarat

Dr. Vikas Karande, *M.V.Sc., Ph.D.*
Assistant Professor,
Department of Pharmacology and Toxicology,
KNPCOVS, Shirwal,
Satara – 412 801, Maharashtra

Dr. Rajinder Raina
Professor
Veterinary Pharmacology and Toxicology,
FVSc and AH (SKUAST-J),
R. S. Pura – 181 102, J&K

Dr. Pawan Kumar Verma, *M.V.Sc., Ph.D.*
Assistant Professor,
Veterinary Pharmacology and Toxicology,
FVSc and AH (SKUAST-J),
R. S. Pura – 181 102, J&K

Dr. Ramesh K. Nirala, *M.V.Sc.*
Assistant professor
Pharmacology and Toxicology,
Bihar Veterinary College,
Patna – 800 014, Bihar

Dr. Hitesh B. Patel, *M.V.Sc., Ph.D.*
Associate Professor
Veterinary Pharmacology and Toxicology,
College of Veterinary Science and Animal Husbandry
SDAU, S.K. Nagar – 385 506, Gujarat

Dr. Ashali Karande, *M.V.Sc.*
Department of Veterinary Medicine
COVAS, Udgir, Latur, Maharashtra

Dr. Nirbhay Kumar, *M.V.Sc., Ph.D.*
Assistant professor
Pharmacology and Toxicology,
Bihar Veterinary College,
Patna – 800 014, Bihar

Dr. Vijeyta Tiwari, *M.V.Sc., Ph.D.*
Assistant Professor,
Department of Pharmacology and Toxicology,
Lala Lajpat Rai University of Veterinary and Animal Sciences (LUVAS),
Hisar – 125 001, Haryana

Dr. N. K. Pankaj, *M.V.Sc., Ph.D.*

Assistant Professor,

Veterinary Pharmacology and Toxicology,

FVSc and AH (SKUAST-J),

R. S. Pura – 181 102, J&K

Dr. V. N. Sarvaiya, *M.V.Sc.*

Assistant Professor

Veterinary Pharmacology and Toxicology,

College of Veterinary Science and Animal Husbandry

SDAU, S.K. Nagar – 385 506, Gujarat

Dr. A. P. Suthar, *M.V.Sc.*

Veterinary Public Health and Epidemiology,

Vanbandhu College of Veterinary Science and Animal Husbandry

NAU, Navsari – 396 450, Gujarat

Dr. Shahid Pravez, *M.V.Sc., Ph.D.*

Associate professor,

Pharmacology and Toxicology,

Faculty of Veterinary Sciences,

Institute of Agriculture Sciences,

BHU, Varanasi– 221 005, UP

Dr. Tariq Ahmad Wani, *M.V.Sc.*

Assistant Professor,

Veterinary Pharmacology and Toxicology,

KCVAS, Amritsar – 143 001, Punjab

Dr. K. Kasturi Devi, *M.V.Sc.*

Assistant Professor

Department of Pharmacology and Toxicology

College of Veterinary Science,

SPVNR TSU VAFS,

Hyderabad – 505 326, Telangana

Dr. Swatantra Kumar Singh, *M.V.Sc.*

Assistant Professor,

Department of Pharmacology and Toxicology,

College of Veterinary Science, NDVSU,

Rewa – 486 001, Madhya Pradesh

Chapter 1

Veterinary Toxicology: An Introduction to the Discipline

☆ *Naveen Kumar*

Toxicology is *"the science of poisons".* In other words, toxicology is the study of poisons and their effects on living organisms. Toxicology involves the knowledge of poisons, including their chemical properties, identification, biologic effects, and the treatment of disease conditions caused by poisons. The term *'toxin'* is used to describe poisons that originate from living cells or organisms and are generally classified as *biotoxins*. Biotoxins are further classified according to their origin as *Zootoxins* (animal origin), *Bacterial toxins* (include *endotoxins* and *exotoxins*), *Phytotoxins* (plant origin), and *Mycotoxins* (fungal origin).

Sources of toxins are mainly of endogenous and exogenous in nature. The endogenous toxins are produced within the body as biochemical by-products which can accumulate in the fat or muscles, whereas the exogenous (external) toxins are ingested or absorbed by the body through water, air, food, drugs *etc.* Moreover, the exogenous poisoning comprises of malicious (intentional), accidental and industrial poisoning.

Veterinary toxicology faces problems related to increase in the use of chemicals and especially to their increased use in animal husbandry and agriculture. In veterinary toxicology, it is important to understand the sources of poisons, circumstances of exposure, diagnosis of the type of poisoning, treatment, and application of management to prevent animals from poisoning.

Scope of Toxicology

People should be concerned about the potentially harmful effects of products they use, medications they take, and the chemicals they are exposed to their everyday lives. Toxicologist helps to understand the potentiality of poison or chemicals and their effects on animals and other living organisms. The toxicologist explores the effects of chemicals on living organisms by using the scientific principles in order to determine the prevalence, quantity and effects of a certain chemical on the environment and human health. The main aim of toxicologists is to examine the threats and hazards surrounding environment and conduct research or experiments to provide protection to animals and humans.

A toxicologist have lucrative career in industry. The toxicologists give information related to substances like food, cosmetics, chemicals or other substances which are safe to use by living organisms. Several organizations, in India and abroad, give lucrative positions and research facilities to toxicologist. Many industries employ toxicologists to assist in evaluating the safety of their products. Toxicologist work as consultants in companies which deal with food, chemical or cosmetic products. Numerous career avenues for toxicologist exist in chemical, food, pharmaceutical, and environment related industries; in teaching and research. Biotechnology and pharmaceutical industries are the largest employers of toxicologists. Toxicologist may work in different areas of toxicology which include academic, clinical, forensic, industrial, pharmaceutical, regulatory *etc.* As there is shortage of toxicologists, qualified and experienced ones get paid well. The salary range is dependent on various factors like the geographical location, organization size and work experience. A toxicologist with postgraduate qualification in veterinary or medical science have bright career in industry. Opportunities in specialized scientific fields depend on background and experiences like immunotoxicology, neurotoxicology, biotechnology and safety pharmacology.

History

- ☆ Earliest humans, who used animal venom and plant extracts for hunting, warfare and remedy.
- ☆ **Ebers papyrus** (about 1500 BC) is among the oldest medical document of ancient Egypt. It contains information of many recognized poisons, including hemlock, aconite (arrow poison), opium, and metals such as lead, copper, and antimony.
- ☆ **Magendie, Orfila, and Bernard**, carried out research in experimental toxicology and laid the groundwork for experimental, therapeutics as well as occupational toxicology.
- ☆ **Magendie**, studied the mechanisms of action of strychnine and "arrow poisons".
- ☆ **Claude Bernard** studied the mechanism of action of carbon monoxide.
- ☆ **Mathieu Orfila** was the first toxicologist to use autopsy material and chemical analysis systematically as legal proof of poisoning. He is considered to be the father of modern toxicology.

★ **Dioscorides**, a Greek physician, classified the poisons into plant, animal and mineral categories.

★ **Theophrastus Phillipus Auroleus Bombastus von Hohenheim (1493-1541)**, a Roman physician (referred as **Paracelsus**), is also considered as the father of toxicology. He described that "all things are poison, only the correct dose differentiates a poison from a remedy". He introduced mercury as the drug of choice for the treatment of syphilis.

Whether a substance is poisonous or not depends on the quantity taken, the species to which it is given, and the route by which it enters the body. For examples:

(a) Small intake of vitamin-A is essential to prevent night blindness, but excess may lead to serious gastrointestinal disorders.

(b) Sugar and salt are nontoxic, but cattle have been poisoned by sugar, and salt poisoning in pigs is well known.

(c) Cobra venom may be drunk with no toxic effect, but it is lethal if administered parenterally.

★ **King Mithridates-VI** discovered an antidote for several venomous reptile and poisonous substances.

★ **Percival Pottrecognisethe** role of soot (polyaromatic hydrocarbon) in scrotal cancer among chimney workers.

★ **Oswald Schmiedeberg** focused on the synthesis of hippuric acid in the liver and the detoxification mechanisms of the liver in animal species.

★ **R. A. Peters, L. A. Stocken, and R. H. S. Thompson**, developed British Anti Lewisite (BAL) as a relatively specific antidote for arsenic.

★ **K. K. Chen**, introduction of modern antidotes (nitrite and thiosulfate) for cyanide toxicity.

★ **C. Voegtlin**, mechanism of action of arsenic and other metals on the SH groups.

★ **P. Muller**, introduction and study of DDT (Dichlorodiphenyl trichloroethane) and related insecticide compounds.

★ **G. Schrader**, introduction and study of organophosphorus compounds (nerve gas agents).

★ **R. N. Chopra** demonstrated that chincona bark extract (quinine) is effective against the malaria parasite. This discovery led to the development of quinine derivatives for the treatment of the disease and the formulation of principles of chemotherapy. He is considered as father of Indian pharmacology for his study on indigenous drugs of India.

★ **William Herschel**, discovered infrared radiation.

☆ **Johann Wilhelm Ritter**, German physicist made the discovery of ultraviolet (UV) ray.

☆ **Heinrich Hertz (in 1887)**, a German scientist, detected first radio waves.

☆ **Wilhelm Rontgen** discovered and named X-rays.

☆ **Henri Becquerel (in 1896)** found that rays emanating from certain minerals penetrated black paper and caused fogging of an unexposed photographic plate, *i.e.*, radioactivity.

☆ **Ernest Rutherford (in 1899)** differentiated alpha rays (α-particles) and beta rays (β-particles).

Classification of Toxicants/Toxicity

I. Toxic compounds are broadly divided into three types

(a) *Physical toxicity-* *e.g.*, coal dust, asbestos, *etc.*

(b) *Chemical toxicity-* *e.g.*, lead, mercury, methyl alcohol, *etc.*

(c) *Biological toxicity-* *e.g.*, bacteria and viruses

II. On the basis of duration of exposure of poison, toxicity may be subdivided into following categories

(a) *Acute toxicity:* Occurs almost immediately (*within hours or days*) after an exposure of chemicals. An acute exposure is usually a single dose received within a 24 hour period. It is measured by the median lethal dose (LD_{50}). LD_{50} is the dose that will kill 50 per cent of a group of animals under stated conditions. *e.g.*, several people were permanently disabled due to acute exposure to methyl isocyanate from an industrial accident in Bhopal, India.

(b) *Sub-acute toxicity:* Duration of exposure to toxicant lasts for a month (*i.e.* generally 28 days of exposure). *e.g.*, Blind staggers in cattle resulting from exposure to seleneferous plants.

(c) *Sub-chronic toxicity:* Duration of exposure lasts for 3 months or less. *e.g.*, industrial exposure to lead over a period of several weeks can result in anaemia.

(d) *Chronic toxicity:* A persistent condition brought on by small repeated exposure of toxicants. The response is measured for a smaller dose over a prolonged period of time, usually for two years. Chronic copper poisoning in sheep is only manifested as haemolytic crisis. Symptoms of bracken fern poisoning may not appear until months after the plant has been ingested.

III. Classification of Poisons on the basis of their relative toxicity

Type of Poison	*Oral LD$_{50}$ Value (in Rats)*
Extremely toxic	< 1 mg/kg
Highly toxic	1-50 mg/kg
Moderately toxic	50-500 mg/kg
Slightly toxic	0.5-5 g/kg
Practically nontoxic	5-15 g/kg
Relatively harmless	> 15 g/kg

IV. Based on damaging organ and system

(a) Gastrointestinal effects: *e.g.*, carbamate, ANTU, abrus, bracken fern, *etc.*

(b) Liver lesions: *e.g.*, Aflatoxin, carbon tetrachloride, paracetamol, phenothiazine, gossypol, *etc.*

(c) Neuromuscular effects: *e.g.*, Botulism, poison hemlock, organophosphates, *etc.*

(d) Bone, teeth, hoof and hair deformities: *e.g.*, Ergot (sloughing of tips of tail, ears, and teats), fluoride (in bone and teeth), arsenic, lead, *etc.*

(e) Kidney Lesions: There are several types of renal damage associated with different toxicants are as follows

    ☆ Degenerative Changes- *e.g.*, chronic organic mercury, chronic thallium, *etc.*

    ☆ Hemoglobinuria- *e.g.*, Crucifers (mustard) and chronic copper toxicity.

    ☆ Hematuria- *e.g.*, Bracken fern, oak, inorganic mercury or cadmium.

    ☆ Oxalates formation- *e.g.*, Ethylene glycol

(f) Lung: *e.g.*, Paraquat.

(g) Retina: *e.g.*, Methanol.

V.   Based on specific lesions

(a) Photosensitization: *e.g.*, Phenothiazines, alfalfa, St. Johnswort, *etc.*

(b) Fever: *e.g.*, Castor bean, oleander, bracken fern and milkweed.

(c) Hemorrhagic syndrome: *e.g.*, Sweet clover, warfarin, radiation, mycotoxins, *etc.*

(d) Abortions and/or Anomalies: *e.g.*, Ergot, fusarium (fungal metabolite) and nitrates. Some compounds may cause birth defects like oak, jimson weed, hemlock and chronic selenium poisoning.

Metabolism (Biotransformation)

The normal metabolic processes of each individual have a limited capacity to adapt to the environmental influences without adverse effects on normal homeostatic mechanisms. Overloading of biochemical processes beyond their ability to adapt can lead to tissue injury whether it is nutrient or other xenobiotic. Every compound has its threshold level of exposure below which there are no toxic consequences but above which dose dependent toxicity is observed. Difference in biochemical process involved in metabolic activation and detoxication also has a major influence on the nature of the toxic response with respect to interspecies differences in sensitivity to toxic chemicals.

Toxicology shares many principles with pharmacology, including process of absorption, distribution, storage, metabolism, and elimination; mechanisms of action; principles of treatment; and dose-response relationships. However, it is not possible to deal with each aspects but it is necessary to discuss some basic principles with their selective examples in the role of detoxication or metabolic activation of xenobiotic.

Detoxification

In general, detoxification of xenobiotic occurs in two phases. In first phase, there is unmasking or introduction of polar functional groups and second phase consisting of conjugation reactions with endogenous substrates (such as glutathione, glucuronic acid, sulphate and amino acid). The primary metabolites commonly undergo second phase of reaction prior to excretion from body, but it is not necessary for all compounds. Some xenobiotics are excreted from body just after first phase of reaction.

A central role in the Phase-I reactions is played by a family of mixed function mono-oxygenase of the cytochrome P450 group. However, other oxygenases may also be involved in first phase oxidation reaction *e.g.*, flavoproteins and cyclo-oxygenase.

The net result of series of reactions is to make the compound more polar (water soluble) and then be excreted from body via urine or bile. Facilitation of excretion of compound prevents accumulation and reduces the toxic effect to the body. See an example (Figure 1.1).

Although these metabolic processes commonly facilitate excretion and reduce the toxicity of non-polar, lipophilic compounds, sometimes the metabolite is highly reactive and more toxic than the parent compounds. In such cases, the compound may be converted into a carcinogen in a process of lethal synthesis.

Lethal Synthesis

In some cases, parent compound which has been taken up by cell is converted into another highly reactive and more toxic compound resulting in death of cell. The metabolite thus produced is an electophile or highly reactive species which can

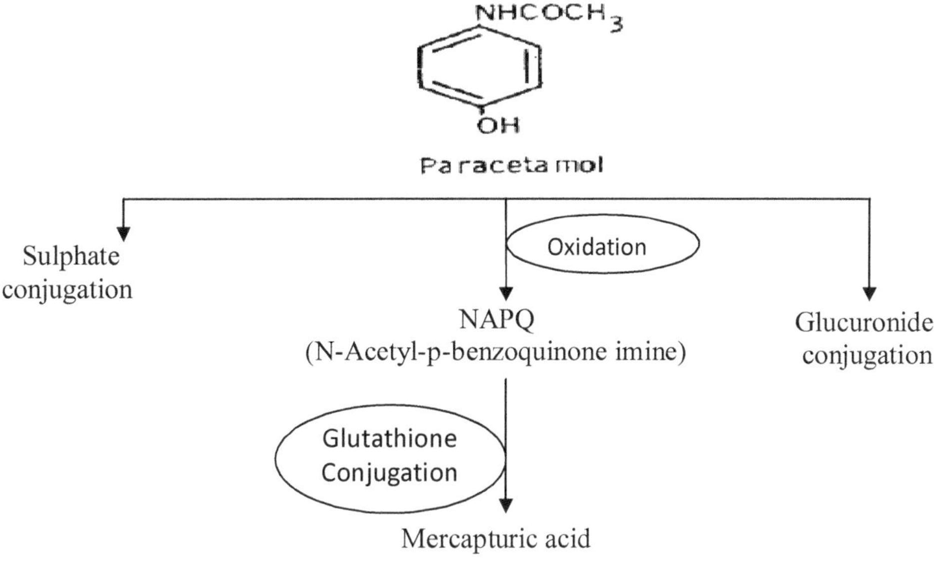

Figure 1.1

undergo covalent bonding with macromolecules such as nucleic acids and proteins. Compounds undergoing covalent bonding with DNA can cause mutagenesis and carcinogenesis. There are several compounds which undergo lethal synthesis. For example:

- ☆ Conversion of fluoroacetate to fluorocitrate- a blocker of aconitase enzyme (resulting in blockade of tricarboxylic acid cycle).
- ☆ Conversion of parathion to paraoxon (a cholinesterase inhibitor), through microsomal oxidation.

Mechanism of Action

Mechanism of toxic action largely involves derangements of the biochemical processes involved in the regulation of cells, tissues and organs. Every organ has a threshold level of exposure of xenobiotic below which there are no toxic consequences but above which dose dependent toxicity is observed. Toxic effect of any chemical is most readily seen when overloading of biochemical process occurs. The most common biochemical processes are congenital metabolic deficiencies, overload of specific enzymes, and inhibition of specific enzymes.

(i) Congenital Metabolic Deficiencies

In case of congenital metabolic disorders, normal dietary concentration of nutrients which are normally well tolerated produce adverse effect *i.e.,* normal dietary constituents may be toxic at relatively low dose. For example, in case of phenylketonuria (PKU) there is genetic deficiency of phenylalanine hydroxylase which is involved in conversion of phenylalanine to tyrosine.

(ii) Overload of Specific Enzymes

In normal condition, there is an equilibrium between circulating haemoglobin and endogenously generated methemoglobin. The methemoglobin is reduced by methemoglobin reductase and only when this mechanism is overloaded *i.e.* when haemoglobin is oxidized to methemoglobin faster than the reduction, does this the circulating methemoglobin level start to rise in a dose dependent way. Initially this condition may be reversible but at higher dose levels anoxia may become apparent. Chronic sub-lethal methemoglobinemia gives rise to splenomegaly and increased haemopoiesis. Methemoglobinemia (met-Hb) is a situation where metabolic overload determines the threshold of toxicity. Methemoglobinemia is a feature of toxicity of aniline, nitrate, hydroxylamines and azo compounds (which are reduced to amines by the gut microflora prior to absorption).

(iii) Inhibition of Specific Enzymes

Many toxic compounds exert their toxic effect to by inhibition of key enzymes involved in cell function regulation. For example, cholinesterase inhibitors which may be naturally occurring (gycoalkaloidsolanin), or synthetic compounds (carbamate and organophosphorus pesticides). The cholinesterase inhibitors block the hydrolysis of acetylcholine which is involved in termination of neurotransmitter action of acetylcholine in synaptic nerve ending in the nervous system and smooth muscle. The death of individual occurs from respiratory failure due to a combination of neuromuscular paralysis and central nervous system depression.

(iv) Binding with Specific Receptors

Chemicals, such as strong acids and bases are toxic simply because they denature proteins and dissolve living tissue. However, some chemical or toxin exerts their toxic effect by binding with specific receptors in cells, thereby disrupting normal biochemical reactions. For example, carbon monoxide interferes with respiration because it has stronger affinity for haemoglobin than the oxygen does, therefore body cannot process sufficient oxygen and death may occur.

Branches of Toxicology

Toxicology is a complex and interdisciplinary subject. Contemporary toxicology is usually divided into following branches:

- ☆ *Clinical toxicology:* It deals with the emergencies occurring due to overdoses of drugs poisonings. It includes identification of the compound, the amount of toxin present in the body, the signs and symptoms caused by the toxin and the control of poisoning.

- ☆ *Forensic toxicology:* It is a branch of forensic science that deals with the study of the cause of death, extracting the toxin from the specimens, amount of poison present and identifying the poison is the main aspect. These studies will lead to the relation between residual levels of the toxins and the cause of death.

☆ *Environmental toxicology:* This branch deals with the study of the toxic effects of various substances on the environment. It includes the effects of water, soil or air pollutants on the living organism and deals with the movement of chemicals in the environment and their residual time.

☆ *Descriptive toxicology:* This refers to the science of toxicity testing of chemicals or agents, usually on animals and their information are correlated for safety evaluation and regulatory requirements.

☆ *Regulatory toxicology:* This deals with analyzing and understanding the data of toxins for risk estimation, the thresholds of solvent vapour in industries and the safe level of drugs for organisms.

☆ *Aquatic toxicology:* The study of effects of toxins on the aquatic organisms. These toxins may be either from manufactured chemicals or can be natural materials. It also includes the effects of toxins at sub cellular level of the individual aquatic organisms.

☆ *Industrial toxicology:* This deals with the study of effects of chemicals released from the industries on the environment and the living organisms. It also deals with the safety of workers of the industry, their exposure to the chemicals, and the safety measures to be taken while working.

☆ *Analytical toxicology:* It is the application of analytical chemistry tools in the quantitative and qualitative estimation of the agents involved in the process of toxicity.

☆ *Toxico-epidemiology:* This refers to quantitative analysis of the toxicity incidences and the use such knowledge in planning prevention and control strategies.

☆ *Eco-toxicology:* This branch deals with effect of toxins at all levels of biological organization from molecular upto the level of ecosystem.

☆ *Molecular toxicology:* Study of determining the modes of action of the toxins and the effect of the toxins at molecular levels. It includes the effects of different toxins on the DNA level, *i.e.,* the mutations that can be caused due to the genes.

Factors Affecting Toxicity

Several factors influence the action of toxicants. In addition to route of absorption and biotransformation, other factors include dosage, physical and chemical nature of the poison, the source of the poison, repeated exposure to the poison, general state of health, species, size, age and sex of the animal.

1. **Physical nature:** The physical state *i.e.,* whether solid, powder or in solution will affect the dose of a poison. Coarsely crystalline arsenic is

slowly absorbed and is relatively less toxic, while finely powdered arsenic is highly toxic.

2. **Chemical nature**: Many substances are readily absorbed from oily solution than from aqueous solution, *e.g.*, insecticides. Chemical nature also is important with regard to toxicity of different toxicants. Yellow phosphorus is a poisonous substance, while red phosphorus is inert, soluble and is excreted unchanged. Compounds containing trivalent arsenic are much more toxic than the pentavalent form. Barium carbonate is intensely toxic than barium sulphate.

3. **The pH of compound and medium:** The pH of toxic compound and medium affect the absorption and distribution of toxicants *e.g.*, if weakly basic strychnine were placed into strong acidic stomach, no systemic toxicity would be observed. However, if the stomach is infused with alkali, most of strychnine becomes un-ionized. Unionized strychnine is readily absorbed and lethal.

4. **Repeated exposure:** Several repeated doses of a poison will produce more serious effect than a single dose. The degree of harmfulness of repeated small doses also depends on whether the poison accumulates in body and its effects are cumulative. Carcinogens are the example of such cumulative and chronic toxicity.

5. **Dosage:** Harmful effect of a toxic compound is largely dependent on the amount of that compound ingested and absorbed into the body.

6. **Species:** There are wide variations in response to a particular poison between different species. For example, cats are susceptible to paracetamol due to deficiency of *glucuronyl S-transferase* enzyme which is involved in the glucuronide conjugation and metabolism of drug. Toxic metabolites may cause methemoglobinemia and hepatotoxicity in animals.

7. **Size, Age and Sex:** In general, the amount of a poison required to produce toxic symptoms is related to the weight of the animals. This relationship between weight and dose may vary between species. Very young and very old animals are usually more susceptible to toxic hazards due to incomplete or less efficient liver biotransforming enzymes and elimination pathways. There are few instances of sex difference in response to poisons in animals. For example, red squill has about twice the toxicity for female rats than for males.

8. **Breed:** Dog breed, such as Bedlington Terriers have tendency to accumulate copper in the hepatocyte, while Collies are more sensitive to neurotoxicity.

9. **General condition of heath:** Debilitated animals are more susceptible to poisons and drugs because their defective resistance and detoxication

mechanisms. For example, patient with hepatic or renal disease are mot susceptible to poisons.

General Approaches to Treatment of Poisoning

In veterinary clinical practice, to provide a diagnosis on poisoning of animals, often multistep approach is needed. There are several components and procedures needed for a good clinical diagnosis and treatment. A veterinarian should perform preliminary diagnostic tests followed by collection and dispatch of appropriate biological samples to toxicology laboratory for detailed investigation. The general approach for diagnosis and management of poisoning cases can be tried as follows:

Approach towards Poisoned Patient

Diagnosis	*Treatment*
☆ History	☆ Emergency medical care:
☆ Physical examination	A. Airway
☆ Recognition of toxic sign and symptoms	B. Breathing
☆ Diagnostic laboratory test	C. Circulation
	☆ Decontamination
	☆ Enhanced elimination
	☆ Fixed or particular therapy

A. Diagnosis

A correct diagnosis is essential before starting specific treatment for poisoning. The various methods of decontamination should be considered in any poisoning cases. The approach should be based on clinical situation of the patient. The first priority is to stabilize the patient and manage life-threatening complications with emergency medical care. Once a poisoning has been identified, methods of poison elimination should be carried out. Specific therapy involves administration of specific antidote when poison is identified. Sometimes, diagnosis and treatment both should be started simultaneously.

i. History

A complete and detailed case history allows the toxicologist to narrow the search for the toxicant which is likely to cause the clinical symptoms. A diagnosis is best made on the basis of the history of suspect poisoning, the occurrence of clinical signs, and the results of laboratory findings.

ii. Physical Examination

Close monitoring of vital signs like heart rate, blood pressure, temperature, ocular findings and respiration are important. Even a direct physical examination can give important diagnostic clues; it should be given low priority compared to the patient stabilization. A physical examination can reveal signs of specific poison. For examples, organophosphates and alcohol poisoning may cause hypothermia, bradycardia, and respiratory depression. Flu like symptoms can be observed with carbon monoxide poisoning.

Neurological Examination

To assessing consciousness in most poisoned animals; alert, painful and unresponsiveness, as simple rapid method can be applies. Seizure is a common presentation in poison or toxins that can induce convulsion.

Some agents that cause seizures include organophosphates, cyanide, chlorinated hydrocarbons, carbamates, lithium, lead and botanicals (*i.e.* water hemlock, strychnine, nicotine). Rotary nystagmus suggests phencyclidine toxicity, whereas horizontal nystagmus is common in alcohol intoxication. Other general neurologic signs include fasciculation (in organophosphate poisoning), rigidity (in tetanus and strychnine), and tremors (in lithium and methylxanthines).

Odours

Some poisons produce characteristic odour that is enough to suggest diagnosis. Important odour that can be observed in poisoned patients are given below:

Odour	Possible Toxicants
Rotten eggs	Sulfur dioxide, Hydrogen sulfide
Garlic	Organophosphates, Arsenic, Selenium, Phosphorus
Bitter Almonds	Cyanide
Freshly mowed hay	Phosgene
Carrots	Water hemlock
Pears	Chloral hydrate

iii. Clinical Finding

Collection of suitable samples for toxicological analysis is critical. Collected tissue or blood sample should be refrigerated and protected from sunlight until the analysis is made. Anticoagulant, EDTA is most commonly used for clinical and analytical purposes. It is important to note the colour and consistency of blood. Chocolate brown blood may indicate methemoglobinemia. High level of urea in the blood might suggest that the animal ingested nephrotoxic agent ethylene glycol. Hair sample is usually helpful for assessing exposure to topical agents such as pesticides. Faeces are suitable for analysis of recently ingested toxicants. The urine sample is helpful in detecting presence of toxicants like paranitrophenol (a metabolite of parathion). Analysis of urine in laboratory may reveal important diagnostic clues.

Colour of Urine	Indication of Toxicant
Orange to red orange	Mercury, chronic lead poisoning
Brown colour	Carbon tetrachloride
Greenish blue	Copper sulphate

B. Treatment

As in any emergency situation. care should be taken for proper ventilation (airway), breathing and to normalize the circulation of poisoned animal. In unconscious animal, go for intubation it may be due to either neuromuscular paralysis or severe respiratory distress: Anesthesia is required for intubation if the animal is conscious. An appropriately sized cuffed endotracheal tube should be placed. Adequate circulation (oxygen delivery) depends on the volume of blood in the vessels and the pumping function of the heart. An early assessment of the electrocardiogram (ECG) will be helpful determining function of the pump. Toxins such as organophosphates, oleander, foxglove, and other cardiotoxic plants directly affect the heart.

Symptomatic treatment should be carried out as soon as possible. Prevent absorption of poisons from the route of entry of toxic substances. Majority of toxin enters through the GI tract. Methods applied for GI decontamination include emesis, gastric emptying or gastric lavage and use of activated charcoal. In cases of ingestion of a caustic liquid such as kerosene, gastric lavage should be avoided because of the risk of aspiration induced lung injury.

Charcoal is a by-product of the combustion of organic compounds such as wood, coconut parts and others. Charcoal is inert, nontoxic, and nonspecific adsorbent that irreversibly binds intraluminal drugs and interferes their absorption. It is particularly effective in binding high molecular weight compounds. In addition, gastric emptying may be beneficial if the ingested drug is not adsorbed by activated charcoal.

Antidotal Therapy

Antidotal therapy should be used carefully, and only after confirmative diagnosis is established. Very limited effective antidotes are available in the market.

Agent (Indication)	Antidote
Organophosphates	Pralidoxime (2-PAM)
Cyanide	Nitrite and Thiosulphate
Arsenic	Dimercaprol (BAL)
Mercury, Lead	Succimer (DMSA)
Iron	Deferoxamine
Colchicine	*Fab* fragments
Ethylene glycol	Fomepizole and Ethanol

Agent (Indication)	Antidote
Carbon monoxide	Oxygen
Paracetamol	N-acetylcysteine (I.V.)
Methemoglobinemia	Methylene blue

Chapter 2

Toxicity of Agrochemicals

✩ *Amita Ranjan and Rakesh Ranjan*

Agrochemicals are chemical compounds (natural or synthetic) used to control or destroy agents (pest or weeds) responsible for loss of agricultural crop production, or have harmful effects on livestock or public health. They comprise two broad groups: (i) Pesticides and (ii) Herbicides. At present more than 150 pesticides are registered with legal application and currently India is the largest pesticide producer country in Asia and ranks 12th in the world. The Green Revolution would not have been possible without availability and widespread application of various agrochemicals. Nevertheless, their increasing production and consumption is posing a serious threat to livestock and public health because many of them persist in the environment, enter into food chain, bio-accumulate in plant/animal/human tissues and produce serious health hazards. Acute toxicity in domestic animals is also common in occurrence. In a survey in Australia, it was found that about 46 per cent cases of toxicity in domestic animals were caused by pesticides. Various agrochemicals, based upon their effect and area of application can be classified into insecticide, fungicide, herbicides and rodenticide (Table 2.1).

According to the regulation, it is essential to write the chemical name and group of agrochemicals, nature of the chemical (caustic/irritant), the specific antidote (if available) and potential to cause toxicity (classification of toxicity potential) on the product leaflet or container. This information is very useful in case of subacute/ acute toxicity arising in animals after their exposure.

Clinical symptoms are often non-specific and confusing, hence history regarding animal and careful examination of premises, grazing pastureland can provide important clue for diagnosis. WHO has classified various hazardous chemicals into different groups on the basis of their hazard potential (Table 2.2).

Table 2.1: Various Types of Agrochemicals and their Utility

Class	Utility/Application
Acaricide	To kill arachnids (spider)
Adjuvant	To improve the efficacy of a insecticide/weedicide
Algicide	To destroy algae
Attractant	To attract insects to a trap
Fungicide	To destroy fungus affecting crop or animal
Growth regulator	Control unwanted plant or insect growth
Herbicide	Destruction of unwanted weeds or plants
Insecticide	To kill insects
Molluscicide	To kill snails and slugs
Repellant	To repel insects and other vertebrate pests
Rodenticide	To kill rodents (rats and rabbits)
Chemical fertilizers	To increase the soil fertility
Preservatives chemicals	For preservation and processing of agricultural product

Table 2.2: Classification of Hazardous Chemicals on the Basis of their Hazard Potential WHO (2009)

WHO Class	Name	LD_{50} for the Rat (mg/kg body weight)	
		Oral	Dermal
Ia	Extremely hazardous	< 5	< 50
Ib	Highly hazardous	5-50	50-200
II	Moderately hazardous	50-2000	200-2000
III	Slightly hazardous	Over 2000	Over 2000
U	Unlikely to present acute hazard	≥ 5000	

I. Pesticides

1. Organophosphorus Compounds

Organophosphorus (OP) compounds are among one of the most common insecticides used in agriculture, animal husbandry, other domestic and industrial purposes. Low cost, wide spectrum, high efficacy and easy availability are reasons behind their widespread use.

Organophosphorus insecticides are esters, amide or other derivates of phosphoric acid and thiophosphoric acid. Unlike organochlorine compounds, they do not accumulate in body fat of man or animals and are rapidly degraded in the environment. In general, they have low mammalian toxicity. Nevertheless, acute toxicity in domestic animals and man due to accidental ingestion of these compounds can occur. Even their prolonged low dose exposure can cause many chronic disorders like cancer, immunosuppression, infertility, peripheral neuropathy and neurobehavioural problems. For these reasons, commercial production of many of these compounds for use as insecticide/pesticide has been banned in the recent past.

Tetraethylpyrophosphate (TEPP) was the first organophosphorus insecticide that was synthesized in year 1854 by Philipe de Clermont. Subsequently, some extremely toxic nerve gases like ethyl N-dimethyl phosphoroamidocyanidate (Tabun) and isopropyl methylphosphonofluoridate (Sevin) were synthesized for their possible use in chemical warfare during the Second World War. Parathion was one of the earliest synthesized OP insecticides with wide application in agriculture. Today, more than 100 organophosphorus compounds are available for use in pest control in agriculture, animal husbandry and public health departments. Some important OP insecticides are listed in Table 2.3.

Table 2.3: Some Important Organophosphorus Insecticides

Aziphos-methyl	Crotoxyphos	Methyl-parathion
Bromophos	Diazinon	Parathion
Carbophenothion	Dioxanthion	Phorate
Chlorpyriphos	Dichlorvos	Ruelene
Chlorhion	Fenitrothion	Trichlorfon
Coumaphos	Malathion	TEPP

General Structure

All OP compounds are esters of phosphoric acid with different combination of attached oxygen, carbon, sulphur, and/or nitrogen. The basic structure of organophosphorus compounds is shown in Figure 2.1. OP compounds can be divided into more than 13 groups on the basis of their chemical structure. However, they all contain a pentavalent phosphorus atom and a characteristic phosphoryl bond (P=O) or thiophosphoryl bond (P=S).

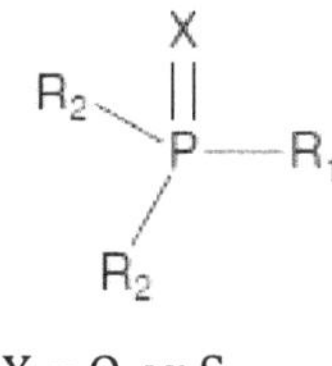

X = O or S

Figure 2.1: General Structure of Organophosphorus Compounds.

Classification

I. OP compounds can be classified into two groups on the basis of their mode of entry.

  (a) Contact poisons: Those compounds which exert their insecticidal action though cutaneous (or cuticle of insects) route are called as contact poisons *e.g.,* parathion, methylparathion, malathion and paraxon.

  (b) Systemic poisons: Those compounds which can enter into the body through gut of the insect and killing them come under this group *e.g.,* dimethoate, mipafox *etc.*

II. On the basis of effectiveness of OP insecticides

  (a) Direct acting compounds: OP compounds that act directly as poison and inhibit cholinesterase enzyme come under this group. For example dichlorvos, diazinon, tricholrfon, chlorothion, chlorpyriphos *etc.*

  (b) Indirect acting compounds: Those OP compounds which in parent form are less/not toxic but are biotransformed into one or more toxic metabolites that are responsible for clinical effects of toxicity come under this group. For example malathion is converted into malaoxon, parathion is converted into paraoxon.

Absorption, Distribution, Metabolism and Elimination

After exposure through oral, dermal, respiratory route (inhalation), OP compounds are absorbed, enter into blood circulation and are distributed in the tissue throughout the body. Inside tissues, they are metabolized either to produce more toxic compound (process known as lethal synthesis) or to produce a compound which is less/not harmful (called as detoxification) and are excreted out from the body. For example malathion is converted into malaoxon (more lethal) as well as malathion monoacid and malathion diacid (less/not toxic).

Mechanism of Toxicity

Organophosphorus compounds inhibit the acetylcholine esterase enzyme (AChE) within the nerve tissue and at the neuromuscular junctions. AChE is responsible for hydrolysis of acetylcholine to produce acetic acid and chlorine. AChE Inhibition leads to accumulation of acetylcholine at the nerve endings and neuromuscular junctions producing characteristic symptoms of parasympathetic (cholinergic) stimulation.

The enzyme AChE has two sites, anionic site and esteratic site (Figure 2.2). Both the sites are vital in hydrolysis of acetylcholine (Ach) molecule. OP compound deactivates them by phosphorylation of serine residue of the active site (esteric sites) of AChE with formation of covalent bond between the enzyme and OP compound. The phosphorylated AChE enzyme is unable to hydrolyse ACh at early stage. Phosphorylated AChE enzyme can be reactivated by AChE reactivators. However, after a lapse of time, dealkylation of the phosphoryl group occurs, making it highly stable and irreversible. This phenomenon is called as "aging" of the AChE

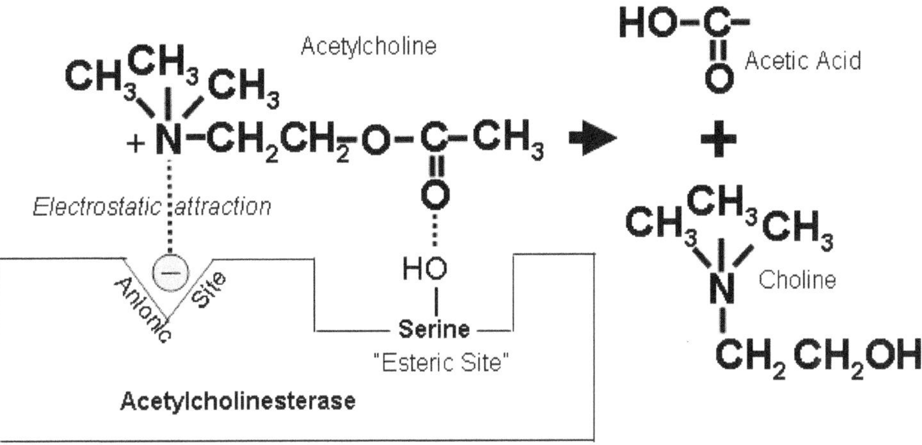

Figure 2.2: Chemical Breakdown of Acetylcholine into Acetic Acid and Choline by AChE.

(Figure 2.3). Mechanism of toxicity of OP compounds and carbamates is similar for insects and mammals.

Clinical Signs

Based upon effects on different receptors, clinical signs of OP insecticide toxicity can be classified into muscarinic, nicotinic and central.

☆ ***Muscarinic receptor associated clinical symptoms*** are first to appear in acute cases and include vomiting, abdominal pain, salivation, lacrimation, frequent urination, diarrhoea, constriction of pupil (miosis/pinpoint pupil), cyanosis and respiratory distress (due to bronchoconstriction and increased bronchial secretion).

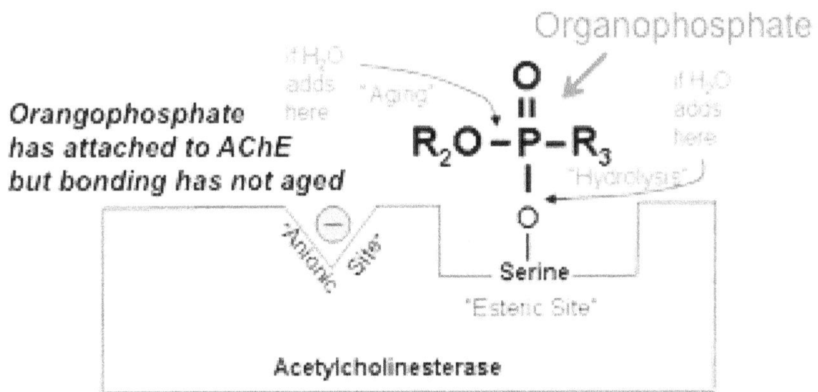

Figure 2.3: Binding of OP Compound on Esteritic Site of AChE and Aging of the Binding.

☆ ***Nicotinic receptor associated clinical symptoms*** include twitching of muscles, tremors, convulsions, seizures and sometimes, generalized paralysis.

☆ ***The central nervous system associated effects*** include apprehension, weakness, ataxia, hypersensitivity and depression.

Excitation and seizures are more common in dogs and cats while depression is more common in ruminants. Other generalized symptoms include restlessness, ataxia, stiffness of the neck, frequent urination and occasionally coma. Death occurs due to respiratory failure (subsequent to respiratory muscle paralysis) or cardiac arrest.

Diagnosis

Diagnosis of OP insecticide toxicity is based upon history, clinical signs and the most specifically upon the activity of AChE activity in blood from a live animal and in brain tissues of a dead animal. More than 70 per cent inhibition of normal AChE activity gives confirmatory diagnosis of OP poisoning. Sometimes, the activity level of AChE may give misleading and inconclusive results. Determining the residue level of various OP compounds in blood or other body fluids by HPLC may be another way for confirmatory diagnosis.

Animals died of OP poisoning show nonspecific lesions in post mortem examination. Pulmonary oedema and congestion may be evident. In rare cases, accumulation of fluid in abdomen and other organs may be present.

Treatment

Line of treatment comprises three basic components:

i. Administration of emetics/cathartics/absorbants to remove ingested poison/minimize absorption of ingested poison.

Administration of emetics or cathartics or gastric lavage is recommended only in monogastric animals when presented within two hours after ingestion of the poison. In ruminants, rumen contents may be evacuated by rumenotomy. Activate charcoal (3-6 g/kg body weight as slurry with water) can be administered orally. If route of exposure is dermal, animal should be washed thoroughly with water.

ii. Administration of anti-muscarinic agents.

Atropine sulphate blocks the muscarinic receptors from Ach. Atropine sulphate treatment (atropinization) can be repeated after every one hour interval till salivation and other muscarinic signs subside and/or pupil dilates. Atropine treatment has no effect on nicotinic signs like muscle twitching and seizures.

☆ In cattle and sheep, it can be given at the rate of 0.5 to 1 mg/kg, with one fourth of the total dose as intravenous infusion (slow) and the remaining through intramuscular or subcutaneous route.

☆ In dogs and cats, atropine can be given at the rate of 0.2 to 2 mg/kg and repeated at every 3-6 hours interval as per the requirement.

☆ For hoses and pig, the dose rate is 0.1 to 0.2 mg/kg IV.

iii. Administration of cholinesterase reactivators.

Pyridine-2-aldoxime methylchloride/iodide (2-PAM) reactivates the AChE inhibited by OP compounds. It combines at anionic site of AChE and exerts a nucleophilic attack on the phosphorus of OP compound producing oximephosphate complex. Oximephosphate complex later on split off and thus AChE is regenerated.

2-PAM is given at the rate of 20-30 mg/kg body weight intravenously as 5 per cent solution. Care should be taken to use only freshly prepared solution and administer slowly as paralysis of respiratory muscles, respiratory failure and death may occur after rapid IV administration. 2-PAM may be repeated after 1 hour at half of its initial dose. It is important to note that 2-PAM is more effective in early stages of the poisoning (within 24 to 48 hours) and does not work after aging of OP compounds.

Diacetyl monoxime (DAM) is another cholinesterase reactivator which is less expensive, have better penetration through blood brain barrier, longer half life and faster in action. The dose rate of DAM is similar to 2-PAM.

iv. Administration of anticonvulsant drugs.

Diazepam or barbiturates administration for controlling seizures should be done with caution, as it may even aggravate the symptoms or result into respiratory arrest and death.

Some Special Effects of OP Compounds

A. OP Induced Delayed Neuropathy/Polyneuropathy (OPIDN or OPIDP)

Some OP compounds, mostly esters of phosphorus containing acids produce delayed neuropathy which is evident in one to three weeks or even months after accidental ingestion in large quantities. Several OP compounds including DFP, mipzfox, TEPP, paraoxon, parathion and haloxon are known to produce OPIDP in man and chicken. The condition is characterized by distal degeneration of long and large diameter mortor and sensory axons of both peripheral nerves and spinal cord. The chicken is the most sensitive animal model. These compounds are weak cholinesterase inhibitors, but inhibit neuropathy target esterase (NTE) enzyme by phosphorylation and dealkylation. Clinical signs include muscle weakness, ataxia and progressive flaccid paralysis of hind limbs.

B. OP Induced Intermediate Syndrome

Ingestion of massive doses of certain OP compounds by human beings is reported to produce a condition clinically characterized by acute paralysis and weakness in areas of several cranial mortor nerves, neck flexors, facial, palatal, proximal limb and respiratory muscles after 24 to 96 hours of poisoning. Here, muscle fasciculations and muscarinic receptor associated symptoms like salivation is completely absent despite marked decrease in AChE activity.

C. Tolerance to Toxicity of OP Compounds

Chronic low dose exposure to OP compounds may result into reduced toxic effects in several animal species. This tolerance to toxicity may develop due to following reasons:

- ☆ Change in number of receptors or decreased affinity of the receptor molecule to OP compound.

- ☆ Presence of some other proteins like albumin or enzymes like carboxylesterases, butyrylcholinesterases *etc.* that can bind or inactivate the OP compound.

- ☆ Rapid hydrolysis of OP compounds inside animal body by enzymes like paraoxonases and somanases.

2. Carbamates

Most of the carbamate (CM) insecticides are esters of carbamic acid (NH_2-COOH). The first CM compound, physostigmine was isolated from calabar beans of the plant *Physostigma venenosum*. Carbaryl was the first synthetic CM compound used as insecticide. Based upon the number of methyl group attached CMs may be classified into two groups: N-methyl carbamates and N,N-dimethyl carbamates (Figure 2.4). However, some carbamate insecticides may contain three methyl groups (like Trimethacarb).

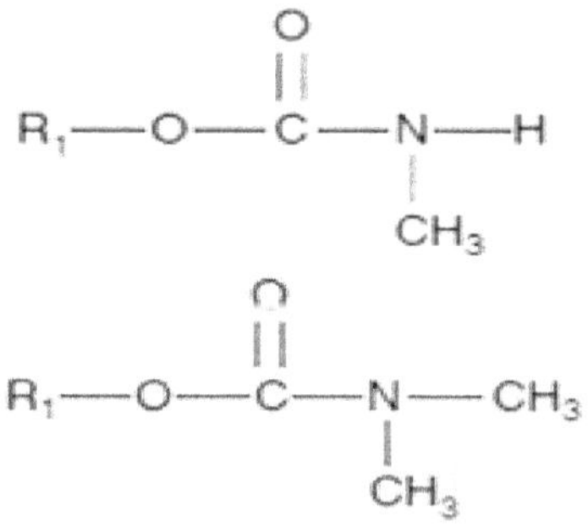

$$R_1-O-\overset{\overset{\textstyle O}{\|}}{C}-\underset{\underset{\textstyle CH_3}{|}}{N}-H$$

$$R_1-O-\overset{\overset{\textstyle O}{\|}}{C}-\underset{\underset{\textstyle CH_3}{|}}{N}-CH_3$$

Figure 2.4: General Structure of Carbamates.

Though appearance of clinical symptoms in carbamate toxicity is faster than OP compound toxicity, the symptoms subsides early because cholinesterase reactivation is spontaneous and rapid. Therefore, carbamate insecticides in general are considered safer than OP insecticides.

Carbamates are rapidly absorbed through skin, lungs and gastrointestinal tract. After absorption, they get rapidly metabolized mainly by glucronide conjugation in liver and are excreted via urine. Carbaryl (Sevin) and Propoxur are two most widely used CM insecticide due to their low mammalian toxicity. Many CM compounds are rapidly degraded in the environment.

Some of the Commonly Used Carbamate Insecticides

☆ Methyl carbamates- Aldicarb, Carbaryl, Propoxur and Metolcarb

☆ Dimethyl carbamates- Carbofuran, Dimetan, Isolan and Primicarb

Mechanism of Toxicity

Like OP compounds, CM produces its insecticidal activity by inhibiting AChE enzyme. Besides, it also inhibit aliesterase enzyme of insects, but inhibition of this enzyme is not lethal for insects. Some differences between mechanism of toxicity of OP and CM compounds are as follows:

a) OP compounds bind only with esteratic site, while CM bind with both anionic as well as esteratic site of AChE enzyme.

b) In general, OP compounds are irreversible inhibitors of AChE, while carbamates are reversible inhibitors of AChE.

c) OP inhibits AChE by phosphrylation while CM inhibits AChE by carbamaylation.

d) Mono-oxime reactivators are effective in OP toxicity, but ineffective in CM toxicity.

Carbamylation is a reversible process; the enzyme-CM bond is spontaneously hydrolyzed and broken. After decarbamylation, the AChE enzyme resumes its functional status but the binding CM compound molecule loses its property and hence become incapable to bind again with other AChE molecule. Therefore, symptoms of CM toxicity do not last long.

Clinical Symptoms

Clinical symptoms and postmortem findings in CM toxicity are similar to OP toxicity. Cholinergic signs are more prominent in acute toxicity, while nicotinic receptor and central nervous system associated signs are more prominent in subacute and chronic toxicity.

Diagnosis

Diagnosis is largely based upon history of ingestion of CM compounds. Laboratory diagnosis on the basis of AChE activity measurement gives erroneous result because it is often normal due to reversible nature of CM-enzyme binding. CM compounds are rapidly degraded in animal tissues, hence estimation of CM residues in biological samples are also inconclusive.

Treatment

Line of treatment is similar to OP compounds, except for oxime reactivators. 2-PAM or DAM should never be given, as they can further aggravate the toxicity. Anticonvulsant drugs like barbiturates and diazepam are also reported to aggravate the CM toxicity. Atropine sulfate in dose as described in OP compound toxicity is recommended for management of CM toxicity.

3. Organochlorine Compounds

Organochlorine compounds (also known as chlorinated hydrocarbons) are mainly used as contact insecticide in agriculture, livestock husbandry and public health sectors. They persist in the environment for long time and can be absorbed through the chitinous cuticle of the insect and have rapid and potent knock-down capacity, hence became highly popular after their discovery. But later on, production and use of many of these compounds was banned due to their bio-accumulative and carcinogenic potential. At present, only lindane and methoxychlor are approved for veterinary use.

Dichlorodiphenyl trichloroethane (DDT) was the first organochlorine compound synthesized by Othmar Zeidler in 1874, but its insecticidal property was discovered by Paul Mueller in the year 1939. He got Noble Prize in the year 1948 for his great discovery. However, it has now been banned for use throughout the world including India due to persistence of its residues in environment and their carcinogenic and bioaccumulative potential in man and animals. Benzene hexachloride (BHC) is another important insecticide of this group. BHC comprises a mixture of eight isomers, among which only gamma isomer, known as "Lindane" has insecticidal property. Lindane is also a banned insecticide due to its known carcinogenic potential. Dicofol and methoxychlor have less toxic potential and persistence in the environment, hence are in use in several countries.

Classification

Organochlorine compound (OC) compounds can be classified into following groups

Group	Examples
Diphenyl aliphatic organochlorines or dichloro-diphenyl ethanes	DDT, methoxychlor, dicofol
Cyclodienes	Aldrin, dieldrin, chlordane, heptachlor, endosulfan
Cyclohexanes	Lindane
Miscellaneous	Kepone, mirax

Absorption, Distribution, Metabolism and Elimination

OC compounds being highly lipid soluble are rapidly absorbed through skin and gastrointestinal tract. However, absorption through respiratory tract is minimal as they are mostly non-volatile compounds (powders). After absorption, they are distributed in liver, kidney, brain and adipose tissues. OC compounds are metabolized through mixed function oxidases (MFOs), glucronide conjugation and sulfonation. Major route of elimination is through digestive tract (biliary excretion), hence enterohepatic recycling is common. Metabolites are largely excreted in faeces.

Mechanism of Toxicity

The diphenyl aliphatic organochlorines such as DDT act by slowing sodium ion influx and inhibiting potassium ion outflow, resulting into excess intracellular deposition of potassium ions in nerve cells. Thereafter, the threshold for another action potential is decreased resulting into premature depolarization of nerve cell. The cyclodienes, in addition to decreasing action potential, act as non-competitive antagonists on the chloride ion channel of the gamma-aminobutyric acid A (GABA$_A$) receptor, thereby inhibiting GABA dependent chloride ion influx into nerve cell. When GABA is inhibited, there is no synaptic down regulation of neurotransmitters like acetylcholine and therefore, cholinergic symptoms appear in toxicity of such compounds. In general, OC compounds are effective insecticide due to its neurotoxic potential.

There are evidences suggesting development of tolerance against OC compounds in some insects. For example DDT resistance due to enzymatic dechlorination of DDT to dichlorodiphenyl dichloroethylene (DDE) was reported in the past.

Clinical Symptoms

Following are important clinical symptoms observed in cases of acute OC compound toxicity:

1. Cholinergic Receptor Related Symptoms

Hypersalivation, vomiting, diarrhoea, abdominal pain and frequent urination. These are non-specific and often confusing symptoms with OP/CM compound poisoning. However, in this case neurological and behavioural symptoms predominates over cholinergic receptor related symptoms.

2. Neurological and Behavioural Symptoms

Anxiety, hypersensitivity, abnormal posture, aggressive behaviour, mania, frenzied behaviour like wall climbing, jumping *etc.,* champing of jaw, twitching of the facial and eyelid muscles, convulsions, seizures and subsequent hyperthermia.

Chronic toxicity of OC compounds is often manifested as hepatic tumour, cancer involving soft tissues, thinning of egg shell in birds *etc.* Cat is the most sensitive animal species for OC toxicity.

Basic differences between the Symptoms of Organophosphate (OP) and Chlorinated Hydrocarbon (OC) Insecticides Poisoning

Symptoms	OP Poisoning	OC Poisoning
Body temperature	Hypothermia	Hyperthermia
Pupil size	Constricted (miosis)	Normal
Salivation	Watery (falling drop by drop)	Frothy type (stick on nose, lip and muzzle)
Movement of the animal	Animal runs in straight direction	Move in circle
Abnormal behavior and posture	Absent	Animal showing abnormal behavior and posture

Treatment

There is no specific antidote available for OC compound poisoning. However, following line of treatment is recommended:

(a) In case of dermal exposure, wash the skin of affected area with water and detergent.

(b) In case of oral exposure of poison

☆ Activated charcoal @ 1-2 g/kg body weight, orally.

☆ Mineral oil, the total oral dose in case of adult cattle is 1-3 litre total doses and in case of dog 5-10 ml is recommended.

Organochlorine compound dissolved in mineral oil, hence their absorption is retarded. However, charcoal or mineral oil is effective only when given within 4 h of pesticide ingestion.

(c) If neurological and behavioural symptoms are intense administer diazepam, phenobarbital or pentobarbital sodium orally or intravenously.

(d) In chronic toxicity or to reduce to amount of OC compound deposited in fat tissues, reduce feed intake of the animal so that adipose tissue is mobilized to meet the nutrient requirement of the body. At this stage, OC compound will also be mobilized and excreted in milk, urine and faeces.

(e) Phenobarbital compounds can induce hepatic microsomal enzyme and hence fasten metabolism and excretion of OC compound.

4. Pyrethrins and Pyrethroids

Pyrethrins are natural chemical compounds with insecticidal property obtained from flowers of the plant *Chrysanthemum cinerariaefolium* (Synonym *Pyrethrum cinerariaefolium; Tanacetum cinerariifolium*). These compounds are highly unstable in the environment, rapidly broken down into non-toxic products when exposed to air, light and heat. Therefore, they have limited use as insecticide. Pyrethroids are synthetic analogues of pyrethrin that are more stable compounds and have wide applicability as insecticide in agriculture, veterinary and public health purposes. In general, they have low mammalian toxicity.

Classification

Based upon the chemical structure, synthetic pyrethroids can be divided into two classes *i.e.*, first and second generation pyrethroids.

1. First Generation Pyrethroids (Type I or non alpha-cyano pyrethroids)

They are esters of chrysanthemic acid and an alcohol, having a furan ring and terminal side chain moieties. *E.g.*, Allethrin, Permethrin, Pyrethrin and Tetramethrin

2. Second Generation Pyrethroids (Type II or alpha-cyano pyrethroids)

They have 3-phenoxybenzyl alcohol derivatives in the alcohol moiety and one or more side chain moiety replaced with a dichlorovinyl or dibromovinyl substitute and aromatic rings. Addition of the alpha-cyano group to the 3-phenoxybenzyl alcohol group is responsible for their increased efficacy as insecticide. *E.g.*, Cypermethrin, Deltamethrin and Fenvelerate

Absorption, Distribution, Metabolism and Elimination

Pyrethroids are lipophilic with low water solubility. Its dermal absorption is very low (equal to nearly 1 per cent). Absorption after oral intake varies from 40-60 per cent, rest are rapidly hydrolyzed and loses its potency in the gastrointestinal tract. After absorption, they are distributed in liver, kidney and other soft tissues with concentration higher in nervous tissue and fat. Metabolism includes action by mixed function oxidases and esterases to produce water soluble compounds that are largely excreted through the urine and up to some extent through faeces.

Mechanism of Toxicity

  ☆ Pyrethrins and pyrethroids slow down the opening and closing of sodium channels, resulting into sustained depolarization of cell membrane. This is particularly more prominent in case of class II pyrethroids.

  ☆ Pyrethroids inhibit the voltage-dependent chloride channels to increase the excitability of the cells in brain, nerve, muscle and salivary glands.

  ☆ Type II pyrethroids, in high concentration also act on GABA-gated chloride channels and calcium ion channels.

  ☆ Some compounds also stimulate nicotinic receptors. Pyrethroids, in general have high cell excitatory effect, but little cytotoxic effect. This property is called as "Knock down effect". Here various ion channels are inhibited, but the integrity of cell membrane is not lost due to absence of any adverse effect on many other cell membrane functions.

Mechanism of toxicity for both insects and mammals are similar, but mammals are less susceptible to pyrethroid toxicity due to following reasons:

  i. The binding of pyrerthroid with sodium channel is stronger at low temperature. Insects have body temperature around 25°C while mammals have body temperature around 37°C.

   ii. Mammalian sodium channels have 1000 times less affinity to pyrethroids than those of insects.

  iii. Mammalian sodium channels recover rapidly from pyrethroid induced depolarization.

  iv. Metabolism and detoxification of pyrethroids in mammals are more rapid and extensive than insects.

Clinical Symptoms

Cats are highly susceptible for pyrethroid toxicity. Clinical symptoms in dogs, cats, cattle and other large animals are similar in case of toxicity by compounds belonging to either of the two groups. Important symptoms are as follows:

☆ ***Muscarinic receptor associated clinical symptoms*** like vomiting, abdominal pain, hypersalivation *etc.*

☆ ***The nicotinic receptor associated clinical symptoms*** include twitching of muscles, tremors, convulsions and seizures.

☆ ***The central nervous system associated effects*** include weakness, prostration, dyspnoea and death.

In rats, the symptoms associated with two groups of compounds are different. In type I compound toxicity, hyperexcitation, tremors and paralysis are major symptoms which are sometimes referred as "T-syndrome" or Tremor syndrome. In group II compound toxicity, choreoathetosis, salivation, weakness and prostration and is referred as "CS-syndrome" or Choreoathetosis-Salivation syndrome.

Treatment

No specific antidote is available for pyrethroids. However, prognosis in subacute cases is good due to low toxic potential and rapid metabolism of pyrethrins inside the body. Following symptomatic treatments should be given as per the intensity of poisoning:

1. In case of dermal exposure, the affected area should be washed with mild soap and water.

2. Adsorbants (like activated charcoal), emetics or purgatives may be given to simple stomach animals if presented within 1-2 h after ingestion of the poison.

3. If seizures or CNS excitement is there, sedatives such as benzodiazepins or barbiturates may be given systematically.

4. If cholinergic symptoms like hypersalivation, vomiting, diarrhoea *etc.* are evident, atropine sulphate should be given.

5. Rodenticides

Rodenticides are chemical compounds used for poisoning or killing rodent pests including rat, mice, squirrel, rabbit *etc.* that are responsible for substantial losses of agriculture and food-stuff during production or storage. Besides, rodents are public health hazard and can transmit many diseases like plague and leptospirosis to man and animals.

An ideal rodenticide should be free from unpleasant taste and smell, should have low toxicity potential in non-target organism, edible for rodents and able to kill the rodents even in low doses. Rodenticide poisoning in domestic and wild animals may arise due to accidental ingestion of rodenticide containing baits, ingestion of rodents died of rodenticide poisoning or malicious poisoning. Incidences are higher in dogs, but usually low in cats, cattle and other domestic animals.

Classification of Rodenticides

Classification of rodenticides can be broadly classified into two groups; anticoagulant and non-anticoagulant rodenticides.

On the basis of their chemical structure anticoagulant rodenticides can be further classified into two groups.

   a. Derivatives of 4-hydroxycoumarin: *e.g.* warfarin, brodifacoum, bromadiolone and Difenacoum

   b. Indane 1-3, dione derivatives: *e.g.* pindone, chlorphacinone and diphacinone.

Furthermore, on the basis of their discovery and potency, anticoagulant rodenticides can be classified into first generation and second generation compounds.

First generation anticoagulant rodenticides were discovered before 1970, have low potency and include dicoumarol, warfarin pindone and valone.

Second generation anticoagulant rodenticides were discovered after 1970, are more potent and include compounds like brodifacoum, bromadiolone, flupropadine, flocoumanafen and diphacinone. Presently, second generation anticoagulant rodenticides are more commonly used.

(A) Anticoagulant Rodenticides

Anitcoagulant rodenticides are rapidly and extensively absorbed after oral intake. In blood, they show strong binding to plasma proteins and therefore, have long half life. They are metabolized by microsome mixed function oxidases (MFO) to form inactive hydroxylated metabolites that are largely excreted through urine.

Mechanism of toxic action includes competitive inhibition of vitamin K epoxide reductase, thereby preventing conversion of vitamin K epoxide to reduced form. The reduced form of vitamin K is required for activation of clotting factors II, VII, IX and X. Ruminants are less susceptible than simple-stomach animals. Drugs inhibiting microbial synthesis of vitamin K in intestine like sulfaquinoxaline may enhance the toxicity.

Clinical signs include epistaxis, dark tarry stools, hematemesis, subcutaneous hematomas, anemia, pale mucous membrane, irregular heart rate, weakness and dyspnea. Animal may die due to shock arising after sustained internal hemorrhage and anemic anoxia.

Diagnosis is based upon several fold increase in blood clotting profile like activated coagulation time, activated prothrombin time and activated partial thromboplastin time. Platlet count may be normal to marginally low.

Treatment of toxicity includes blood transfusion, and administration of Phytonadione (Vitamin K_1) by oral/intramuscular/subcutaneous route (not by intravenous route) at the rate of 2 to 5 mg/kg body weight. Vitamin K administration is continued for few days during the convalescent period.

Warfarin

The chemical name of warfarin is (RS-4-Hydroxy-3-(3-oxo-1-phenylbutyl)-2H-chromen-2-one. It was originally discovered from spoiled sweet clover (*Melilotus-spp.*) based animal feed. It is rapidly detoxified in the liver. Its long-term use as rodenticide is limited as rodents quickly develop resistance to it. Dogs, pigs, cats and horses are susceptible to warfarin toxicity. Warfarin, act as vitamin K antagonist. Massive internal hemorrhage starts 2 to 5 days after ingestion of the poison or poisoned rodents. Clinical signs of toxicity include epistaxis, hematoma formation, bloody discharge from natural orifices, dyspnea, exercise intolerance, weakness and collapse. Diagnosis, as described above is based upon profiling of blood coagulation factor. Treatment includes blood transfusion, vitamin K_1 analogue administration, sedative/tranquilizer administration to calm down the animal and reduce the oxygen demand.

(B) Non-anticoagulant Rodenticides

1. Phosphides of Zinc/Aluminium/Calcium

Zinc (or aluminium or calcium) phosphide is a popular rodenticide because of low cost and high efficacy. They are unstable compounds and are degraded rapidly in acidic or moist environments. Dog and cat may show signs of acute toxicity 0.5 to 4 hours after ingestion of either rat baits directly or poisoned rodents. In acidic gastric environment, phosphides are hydrolyzed to release phosphine gas which is rapidly absorbed across the mucous membrane.

Mechanism of toxic action includes direct corrosive/irritant action of phosphide salts on gastrointestinal and respiratory system and inhibition of Cytochorme C oxidase enzyme. However, the role of Cytochorme C oxidase inhibition in phosphide toxicity is not clear.

Toxicity is very much dependent upon pH of the stomach. If the poison is ingested when gastric acid secretion is high and pH is low (after food intake) the toxicity is more, but when ingested empty stomach (when pH is high or gastric acid secretion is low), the toxicity is low. The lethal dose for most animals varies between 20 to 50 mg/kg body weight.

Clinical signs of toxicity include vomiting, depression, tremors and weakness. In ruminants, bloat, hypersthesia, seizures and CNS excitement may be evident. Signs of abdominal pain and hypersalivation may also be evident in horse and dog. Acetylene (or dead fish) like odour (due to phosphine gas) is present in gastric contents of dead animals.

Treatment primarily include oral administration of activated charcoal. Intravenous fluid and bicarbonate therapy should be given to prevent acidosis. Blood calcium level should be monitored and intravenous calcium borogluconate should be given. Gastric protectants may be given in dogs and cats to safeguard GIT from irritant action of the poison.

2. Bromethalin

It was developed as an alternative for use in warfarin-resistant rats. Dog and cat may suffer from toxicity after accidental or malicious poisoning. It is rapidly absorbed after oral intake. Bromethalin uncouples oxidative phosphorylation and inhibit sodium pump resulting into cellular edema, cell swelling and degeneration.

Clinical signs of acute toxicity include hyperexcitability, paddling, hyperesthesia, muscle tremor and pyrexia. In subacute poisoning, CNS depression, loss of reflexes, ataxia and posterior paralysis appear as major clinical symptoms.

Diagnosis is based upon history, clinical symptoms, abnormality in electroencephalogram and increase in CSF pressure.

Treatment options include oral administration of adsorbants like activated charcoal or emetics. Intravenous mannitol may be given to reduce the CSF pressure. Phenobarbital or benzodiazepine compounds may be given if seizures or CNS excitement is evident.

3. Sodium Fluoroaceate and Fluoroacetamide

Sodium fluoroacetate (Compound 1080) and fluoroacetamide are colourless, odourless and tasteless salt soluble in water. It is highly toxic to rodents as well as other vertebrates, particularly carnivores including dog and cat. In some countries, it is also used as bait for fox control. The toxic doses for most domestic mammals is less than 1 mg/kg, while for rodents, the lethal dose is 5- 8 mg/kg body weight. Toxicity in dogs and cats may also arise after ingestion of poisoned rodents.

Sodium fluoroacetate and fluoroacetamide are rapidly absorbed from GIT. They replace acetyl-coenzyme A and combine with oxaloacetic acid to form fluorocitrate. Fluorcitrate inhibits aconitase in the citric acid cycle (TCA or Kreb's cycle), thus inhibits cellular respiration and energy production.

Clinical signs appear usually within 2 hours after ingestion and include restlessness, vomiting, diarrhoea, frequent defecation, urination, hyperirritability, frenzied running, barking, frothing from the mouth and nostrils, dyspnea and seizures. In cats, cardiac arrhythmia and abnormal vocalization is observed. In horses and cattle, sudden death due to cardiac arrest occurs.

Diagnosis is based upon history, clinical signs and laboratory evidence of hyperglycemia, acidosis and elevated citrate levels in blood.

Treatment includes administration of activated charcoal or emetics or gastric lavage, if animal is presented soon after ingestion of the poison.

- ☆ Thiobarbiturate or diazepam may be given if seizures or CNS excitation is there.
- ☆ Glycerol monoacetate @ 0.55 g/kg given intramuscularly at hourly interval until a total dose of 2-4 g/kg is achieved.
- ☆ Ethanol (50 per cent) and acetic acid (5 per cent) orally @ 8 ml/kg may help reducing conversion of fluoroacetate to fluorocitrate.

4. Alfa Napthyl Thiourea (ANTU)

ANTU have low toxicity potential in non-target species, but may induce toxicity in dog and cat after ingestion of rodent, died of ANTU toxicity.

Mechanism of toxic action includes increased capillary permeability of pulmonary blood vessels resulting into pulmonary oedema, impaired pulmonary oxygenation, anoxia, cyanosis and death. Clinical signs of toxicity include irritation of gastric mucosa hence induces vomiting in dog and cat when ingested empty stomach. Other clinical signs are hypersalivation, abdominal pain, frequent urination, dysponea, snoring, coughing, tachycardia, cyanosis of mucous membrane, incoordination, convulsions and death. Massive pulmonary oedema and hydrothorax is evident in animals died of the ANTU poisoning. Diagnosis is based upon history and clinical signs.

Treatment includes use of emetics and sedatives, oxygen therapy and diuretics to relieve pulmonary oedema. 1-ethyl-1-phenyl thiourea acts as a competitive antagonist of ANTU hence may be tried as antidote.

5. Red Squill

Red squill contains a cardiac glycoside known as scilliroside. It is obtained from sea onion (*Urginea maritima*) plant. Clinical signs of red squill toxicity include hyperaesthesia, incordination, excitation, convulsions and death. In high doses, death occurs due to cardiac arrest without showing any clinical signs. Post mortem lesions are non-specific including congestion and hemorrhages in stomach, intestine, liver, kidney and lungs. Diagnosis is based upon history and clinical lesions. Symptomatic treatment is suggested as no specific antidote is available.

II. Herbicides

Herbicides are chemical compounds used for killing or controlling growth of weeds or unwanted plants in agricultural field, roadside, residential lawns or industrial sites. Herbicides account for nearly 60 per cent of all pesticide sales in USA. They are largely used in countries where intensive and highly mechanized agriculture is practiced. Together with fertilizers and pesticides, herbicides improve the plant growth, and made an important contribution to increase yields. However, accidental ingestion of these chemicals in large doses or grazing of freshly sprayed pasture or consuming hay prepared from treated plants may result into toxicity in animals. Most herbicides, in general have low mammalian toxicity hence incidence of herbicide toxicity is also low.

Classification

Based upon the chemical structure, herbicides can be broadly classified into two groups:

a. Inorganic Herbicide

Inorganic herbicides are old generation herbicides, rarely used in modern agriculture practices. It includes arsenicals (sodium arsenite), bittern, copper sulphate, chlorates, ammonium slfamate *etc.* Most of them are non-selective in action and have high mammalian toxicity potential.

b. Organic Herbicide

They are modern herbicides selectively effective against weed and have low environmental and mammalian toxicity potential. Organic herbicides can be further classified into different categories on the basis of their chemical composition.

On the basis of application, herbicides can be classified into pre-emergent and post-emergent herbicides. Pre-emergent herbicides are incorporated in soil to prevent germination of unwanted plants. Post emergent herbicides are applied directly to growing plants to destroy or kill them.

Based upon the chemical composition, herbicides can be classified into several groups like phenoxyaliphatic acid derivatives, bipyridinium compounds, dinitro compounds, triazines, chlorinated aliphatic acid derivatives, urea derivatives, carbamates, substituted aliphatic acids *etc.* Some important groups of herbicides and their toxicity in animals are as follows:

1. Phenoxyaliphatic Acid Herbicides

Examples are 2,4- D, MCPA, Silvex, 2,4,5-T, MCPB, 4-CPA *etc.*

They are chlorinated phenoxy derivatives of fatty acids and make a major group of organic herbicides. They are rapidly absorbed from stomach and intestine, but dermal absorption is poor. After absorption, they are rapidly distributed into blood and soft tissues. Besides causing direct toxic action, these herbicides are also responsible for increase in the nitrate content of certain plants and increase palatability of certain toxic plants like Sudan grass and larkspur. Cattle and dogs are susceptible for toxicity of phenoxy herbicides. Mechanism of toxic action include uncoupling oxidative phosphorylation, increase in number of hepatic peroxisomes, suppression of ribonuclease synthesis and effect on muscle membrane. The clinical symptoms are related to gastrointestinal and neuromuscular system and include anorexia, vomiting, diarrhoea, ruminal atony, ulceration of oral mucosa, bloat, depression, muscle weakness, ataxia, tremors and changes in electrocardiogram. Treatment includes administration of activated charcoal or emetics, symptomatic treatment of gastrointestinal and neuromuscular symptoms.

2. Dipyridyl/Bipyridinium Herbicides

E.g. paraquat and diquat.

They are water soluble, non-volatile compounds, rapidly and completely degraded in soil by bacterial activity and by sunlight too. They are broad spectrum, rapid acting contact (desiccant) herbicides and are extensively used in cotton and potato crops. Absorption from gastrointestinal tract (20 per cent approx) as well as through skin (about 10 per cent) is poor. Absorbed compound is distributed widely in soft tissue, but concentration of Paraquat in lungs is 10 times higher than other soft tissues. There is excessive generation of reactive oxygen species inside cells leading to oxidative degeneration and necrosis. The toxicity may be chronic or acute in nature.

In acute toxicity, vomiting, depression, ataxia, dyspnea and seizures appear first, followed by respiratory signs including tachypnea, dyspnea, moist rales and cyanosis. In subacute or chronic toxicity, progressive pulmonary fibrosis and respiratory distress are important clinical signs.

Diagnosis is based upon radiographic changes in lungs, history of exposure to pesticides and clinical symptoms. Post-mortem lesions include pulmonary congestion, hemorrhage, emphysema and broncho-dilatation. Sometimes, spongy degeneration of cerebral white matter is also evident.

Treatment includes oral administration of activated charcoal or Bentonite or Fuller's earth or clay-based adsorbants. In case of dyspnea, assisted ventilation may be given, but oxygen therapy is contraindicated as it may further enhance the free radical generation and tissue damage. Antioxidant vitamins including ascorbic acid and riboflavin may be helpful. Acetylcysteine may serve as substitute for glutathione in the reduction of free radicals. Diuretics may help in reducing pulmonary oedema and renal damage. Tranquilizers and sedative may be needed when nervous signs predominate or to calm down the animal.

3. Dinitro Compounds

E.g., Dinitro ortho cresol (DNOC) and dinitrophenol.

Mechanism of toxic action of dinitro herbicides include uncoupling of oxidative phosphorylation and thereby enhancing cellular heat production. Hyperthermia develops in dinitro compound toxicity. In ruminants, dintro compounds are degraded in diamine compounds in rumen, inducing methaemoglobinemia. Rigor mortis develops quickly in animals died of the poisoning.

Diagnosis is based upon history, clinical symptoms and post-mortem lesions. No specific antidote is available. Hyperthermia may be alleviated by application of ice-pack or cold water but use of antipyretics is contraindicated. Sedatives may be required to calm down the animal. Methylene blue may be given in ruminants to control methaemoglobinemia.

4. Triazenes/Heterocyclic Compounds

Compounds of this group include Atrazine, Propazine, Cyanazine and Simazine.

Atrazine (6-chloro-N-ethyl-N'-(1-methylethyl)-1,3,5-triazine-2.4-diamine) is the most widely used herbicide of this group. It is a white crystalline powder and used on sugarcane crops and on roadway grasses, residential lawns and other public places. Atrazine is recognized as an endocrine disruptor that alters the reproductive cycle and induces mammary tumors in rats. Chronic toxicity is reported to increase the age of puberty and sexual maturity in rats. Atrazine have low mammalian toxicity potential. Other compounds of this group like prometone are more toxic and induce pulomonary oedema and gastric and intestinal haemorrhages. In acute toxicity, hypersalivation, weakness, ataxia and posterior paralysis appear 2-3 weeks after exposure of the poison. No specific antidote is available, hence symptomatic treatment is recommended.

III. Fungicides

Fungicides are agents used to inhibit or kill fungi. They are extensively used in agriculture, domestic and industry purposes for the following purposes:

   i. Protection of tubers, fruits, vegetables, seed grains.

   ii. Protection of ornamental flowers, trees, cereal crops and grasses.

   iii. Preservation of wood, suppression of mildews that attack painted surface and control of slime in paper pulps.

   iv. Protection of household carpet and fabrics.

   v. Treatment of fungal diseases in animals.

Annual consumption of fungicides across the world is estimated to be 500 million pounds. In general, mammalian toxicity potential of majority of modern fungicides is moderate to low, but many of them are responsible for dermal sensitization, irritant injuries to skin and mucous membranes and chronic toxicities including hepatic and renal damage and carcinogenesis.

Elemental sulphur and lime sulphur have long been used as fungicides. They rarely cause toxicity, except when used in micronized form. Cattle, sheep and goat are mostly affected and show gastric, neurological and respiratory symptoms.

Toxicity potential of a given fungicide also varies with animal species. Some fungicides like copper sulphate, chlorothalonil and captan are highly toxic for fish and honey bees. Mercurial fungicides are highly toxic to birds. Moreover, fungicides

Table 2.4: Classifications of Fungicides on the Basis of their Chemical Nature

Chemical Class	Example	Major Toxicity and Treatment (if any)
Halogenated substituted monocyclic aromatics (Substituted benzenes)	Chlorothalonil	☆ Irritation to skin and mucous membranes, very toxic for fish (gill damage and anemia). React with –SH group ☆ Wash the skin with soap and water.
	Hexachlorobenzene (HCB) (Note: it is different from hexachlorocyclohexane, gamma isomer, which is known as Lindane)	☆ Liver enlargement, neurological changes, immunosupression, teratogenic and carcinogenic effects. ☆ Administer activated charcoal
	Dicloran	☆ Toxic to birds (kidney, liver and hematopoietic system damage)
	Pentachlorophenol (PCP; used as wood preservative)	☆ Embryotoxic and fetotoxic (not teratogenic), irritation to skin and mucous membrane, cause energy depletion by inhibiting Na^+ -K^+ ATPase and thereby uncoupling oxidative phosphorylation. ☆ In acute toxicity pyrexia, increased respiration, glycosuria, cardiac and muscular collapse and death. ☆ Anemia in chronic toxicity.
Copper compounds	Copper acetate, copper ammonium carbonate, copper lime dust, copper sulphate, Bordeaux mixture	☆ Powder or dust of copper compound is irritant and corrosive, systemic toxicity is observed after oral intake.
Organomercurial compounds	Methyl mercury, methoxyethyl mercury and phenyl mercuric acetate	☆ Nervous excitement, ataxia and convulsions.
Thiophthalimide (Chloroalkyl thiodicarboximides)	Captan, Captafol and Folpet	☆ In general, have low mammalian toxicity. ☆ Susceptibility: Fish > Sheep > Cattle. ☆ Symptoms in sheep include anorexia, hypothermia, depression, diarrohea, weight loss and death.
Benzimidazoles	Benomyl, carbendazim, fuberidazole and thiophanate-methyl and thiabendazole.	☆ Toxicity may arise due to ingestion of these compounds, hepatotoxic, embryotoxic and teratogenic. Sometimes nervous symptoms like tremors, hypersalivation, convulsions may appear

Chemical Class	Example	Major Toxicity and Treatment (if any)
Strobilurin fungicides	(Zoxystrobin, Picoxystrobin, Pyraclostrobin, Trifloxystrobin) New group of fungicides used in agriculture to kill mildews, molds and rusts.	☆ Irritant to skin and mucous membrane, inhibits mitochondrial respiration by blocking electron transport chain. ☆ In general, have low mammalian toxicity. Treatment: symptomatic
7. Carbamic acid derivatives	a. Dithiocarbamates: Metam, Ferbam, Thiram and Ziram	☆ Low to moderate mammalian toxicity except for Nabum (disodium ethylene bis dithiocarbamate).
	b. Ethylene bis dithiocarbamates: Mancozeb, Maneb, Nabam, Metiram and Zineb	☆ Thyroid hypertrophy and hyperplasia (sustained high TSH). Metabolized and eliminated rapidly through urine and faeces. ☆ Metam sodium decomposes in water to yield methyl isothiocyanate, an extremely irritating gas producing severe lung irritation (edema). ☆ Thiram is hepatotoxic and produces nervous symptoms like listless behaviour, convulsions, anorexia and death.
Triazoles compounds	Triadimefon, Myclobutanil, Propiconazole, Flutriafol	☆ Low systemic and dermal toxicity. In mice and rats causes hepatocyte hypertrophy, hyperactivity, excitement *etc.*
Cadmium (Cd) compounds	Cadmium chloride, Cadmium succinate, Cadmium sulphate (wood preservative)	☆ After ingestion, vomiting, diarrhoea, abdominal pain *etc.* ☆ After inhalation, Cd compounds produce respiratory distress, pulmonary oedema and penumonitis. ☆ In chronic toxicity, hepato-renal damage, proteinuria, anemia and jaundice and COPD (Chronic obstructive pulmonary disease). ☆ Diagnosis is based upon estimation of Cd concentration in blood, urine and other body fluids. ☆ Treatment mostly symptomatic, chelation therapy with calcium disodium EDTA, oral-adsorbants, fluid therapy, manage hepato-renal damage associated changes.

are frequently used in combination with other pesticides and solvents that enhances the toxicity potential of the fungicide.

Classification

Broad classification, example, major mechanism of toxic action and specific treatment options of different fungicides are given in Table 2.4.

Toxicity of some Hazardous Fungicides

1. Copper Compounds

Several copper compounds including sulphates, acetates, oxides and oxychlorides are used as antifungal agents for wood preservation and in fabric industry. Bordeaux mixture, an old fungicidal agent is a mixture of hydrated lime and copper sulphate.

Cupric sulphate pentahydrate (Copper sulphate/Blue vitrol) is used to control fungal diseases like mildew, life spots and blights in horticulture. Besides, it also has algaecidal and molluscicidal properties. Copper toxicity may be acute or chronic. Sheep appears to be highly susceptible for copper toxicity. Copper compounds inhibit G6-P-D, NADPH and glutathione reductase enzymes resulting into damage of RBC membrane and hemolysis.

Clinical symptoms of acute poisoning include vomiting, hypersalivation, greenish diarrhoea and abdominal pain. Sometimes, nervous symptoms like convulsions and paralysis are also recorded. In chronic poisoning liver damage, anemia, hematuria, icterus, hepatomegaly and anorexia are common symptoms. Diagnosis is based upon history and estimation of whole blood and serum copper concentrations.

Treatment options include administration of activated charcoal, sedatives and other drugs on the basis of clinical symptoms. In chronic poisoning, daily administration of dimercaprol @ 2-4 mg/kg by intramuscular route for 2-3 days may be tried. Another antidote disodium calcium EDTA @ of 40-50 mg/kg by intravenous route once daily for 2-3 days may be tried. Oral administration of ammonium molybdenate and sodium thiosulphate is also recommended in chronic copper toxicity.

2. Organomercurial Compounds

Organomercurial compounds inhibit protein synthesis by inhibiting sulfhydryl group of enzymes involved in the transfer of amino acids. Organomercurial fungicides can be broadly divided into three groups:

A. *Methyl Mercury Compounds*

e.g., Methyl mercury (hydroxide/acetate/propionate/pentachlorophenate/ quinolinolate)

B. Methoxyethyl Mercury Compounds

e.g., Methoxyethyl mercury (acetate/chloride)

C. Phenylmercuric Acetate

e.g., Agrosan, Unisan Phenyl mercury ammonium acetate

Organomercurial compounds inhibit protein synthesis by inhibiting sulfhydryl group of enzymes involved in the transfer of amino acids.

The organomercurial compounds are absorbed by all routes and can accumulate in body tissues to produce cumulative toxicity. Methyl mercury compounds are poorly excreted from the body and tend to accumulate in muscle, brain, erythrocytes and other soft tissues. However, phenylmercuric acetate is readily excreted via the kidney and hence less likely to accumulate in body tissues. Toxicity in animals may develop either directly by ingestion of organomercurial compounds or by chronic intake of low doses of these compounds through contaminated meat or fish meal.

Diagnosis is based upon estimation of mercury concentration in blood and body tissues. Toxicity is usually chronic and exhibited as nervous system involvement like blindness, abnormal behaviour, excitation, incoordination, ataxia and convulsions. Symptoms once developed are largely irreversible. However, dimercaprol in a dose similar to described in copper toxicity may be tried. Penicillamine @ 15-50 mg/kg also help in elimination of organomercurial compounds from body tissues.

3. Chlorothalonil

This belongs to halogenated substituted monocycylic aromatic fungicide. Topical exposure leads to skin irritation, eczema, pustules, ulceration and keratinisation. It is a immunotoxic, hepatotoxic and neurotoxic compound. Clinical cases of toxicity are presented with CNS signs like incoordination, ataxia, prostration, convulsions and death. Calf, dog, cat and rat are highly susceptible for toxicity.

4. Hexachloro-benzene (HCB)

It accumulates in adipose tissue and may induce chronic toxicity. It inhibits chytochrome P 450 and conjugate enzymes. Chronic toxicity is manifested as hepatomegaly, focal alopecia, eruptions, pigmented scar and chronic weight loss. Sometimes, nervous signs including irritability, ataxia and tremors may appear. The compound also has immunotoxic and teratogenic effects in laboratory animals. Acute toxicity in cattle and sheep suggest pyrexia, increased breathing rate, tremors, convulsions and death.

Line of Treatment for Fungicide Toxicity in Animals

☆ In case of recent oral exposure to large doses of fungicides administration of emetics, gastric lavage or activated charcoal is recommended.

☆ In case of dermal exposure, wash the exposed area with plenty of water and soap.

- ☆ If nervous excitement is there give phenothiazine tranquilizers. But these compounds should not be used when there is depression or the animal is unconscious.

- ☆ Administer balanced electrolyte solution. Give oxygen therapy if there is respiratory distress.

- ☆ If fever is present, antipyretics are recommended.

- ☆ Specific antidotes, if available should be given at recommended doses. Dimercaprol (BAL) or sodium thiosulphate may also be given in recommended doses.

Urea Toxicity

Urea is used as fertilizer in agriculture and as a low cost protein substitute in feed for ruminants. Toxicity of urea in ruminants occurs after accidental ingestion of excess urea either due to improper mixing in feed or intake of fertilizer as such. Tolerance develops after low dose urea intake for long time, but tolerance is reduced by starvation and low protein diet. Toxicity signs appear when ruminants are fed urea @ 20 g/kg body weight or more. Simple stomach animals like horse and pigs can tolerate high doses of urea without showing any clinical sign of toxicity.

Mechanism of Toxic Action

Urea is broken down into ammonia due to action of urease enzyme present in the rumen (Figure 2.5). The ammonia released is rapidly absorbed in the rumen. The intensity of clinical symptoms correlates with the ammonia level in blood.

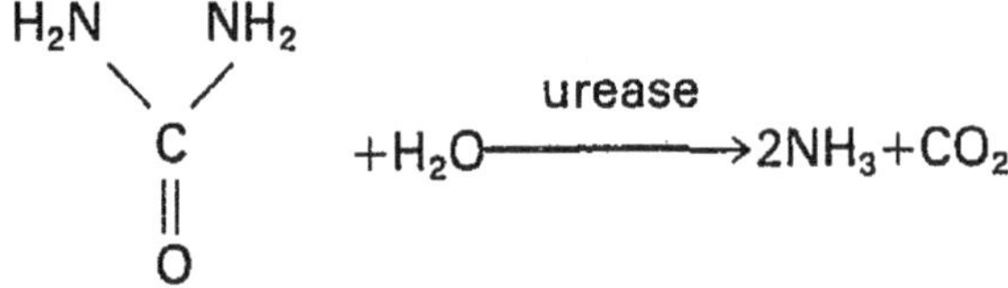

Figure 2.5: Action of Urease Enzyme on Urea.

Clinical signs appear within 10 to 20 minutes after urea intake and include frothing from mouth, hypersensitivity, aggression, muscle tremor, incoordination, bloat, abdominal pain, difficult breathing, weakness, recumbancy and death. Death is supposed to occur due to respiratory arrest. Non-specific post mortem lesions like generalized congestion and hemorrhage in visceral organs and pulmonary oedema are recorded in animals died of urea toxicity.

Diagnosis is based upon history, clinical signs and examination of rumen fluid which is high in pH (7-8) and have ammoniac odour. Blood ammonia concentration in affected animals reaches up to 0.7 - 0.8 mg/dl.

Treatment includes administration of a weak acid like vinegar (2-4 litre in an adult cattle and 0.5 to 1 litre in an adult sheep). This helps reducing absorption of ammonia from rumen. Evacuation of rumen content by rumentomy is the most effective life saving option in urea toxicity. In most cases of acute urea toxicity animals die before diagnosis or prior to treatment. Restoration of ruminal microflora (by cud transfer/administration of probiotics/rumenotorics) and appetite of animal is to be undertaken in remaining animals.

Chapter 3

Toxicology of Mineral Elements

Mineral elements are essential for survival, production and reproduction of animals. Many of them are essential for metabolism and synthesis of body constituents. However, when ingested in excess, they may cause either acute or chronic toxicity. Acute toxicity occurs when ingested in large doses over a short time span, whereas chronic toxicity occurs after exposure to low doses over prolonged period. Some minerals are required in substantial amount for which body has wide tolerance (*e.g.*, sodium and iron), whereas some metal is required in much smaller amounts, and for which the body has a quite narrow tolerance (*e.g.*, copper). Some minerals do not have any role in body metabolism and are toxic even in very low doses (*e.g.*, lead and mercury).

Metal toxicosis due to heavy metals are not uncommon in veterinary. Such toxicity can be effectively enounter by use of their particular antagonist. Metal antagonist competes with their reactive groups for metal, thereby prevents their toxic effects and enhances their excretion. Such antagonists are often referred as chelating agents. Chelators have ability to form complexes with metals and thereby prevent the binding of metals to body ligands. The stability of chelates varies with the metal and the ligand atoms. For examples, lead and mercury have greater affinities for sulphur and nitrogen than for oxygen ligands. The effectiveness of a chelating agent for treatment of metal poisoning depends on several factors, such as relative affinity of the chelator for the heavy metal as compared to essential body metals, distribution of the chelator in the body as compared with the distribution of the metal, and the ability of the chelator to mobilize the metal from the body which one is chelated.

Common properties of an ideal chelating agent:

a. Chelating agent should be highly soluble in water for better excretion

b. Resistance to biotransformation

c. Ability to reach sites of metal storage

d. Capacity to form nontoxic complexes with toxic metals

e. Low affinity for Ca^{2+} is also desirable, because Ca^{2+} in plasma is readily available for chelation, and a drug might produce hypocalcaemia despite high affinity for heavy metals

f. The greater affinity for the metal than that for the endogenous ligands.

g. Ability to retain chelating activity at the pH of body fluids

Preventive Measures for Toxicity

i. Surveillance

This is the backbone of any effective preventive programme. A heavy metal toxicant surveillance programme has some essential factors that must be considered before undertaking any control measure. These factors are:

☆ The determination of heavy metal toxicants in food/feed.

☆ The determination of food/feed consumption.

☆ The estimation of total load of heavy metal contaminant from all sources of exposure, including air, water, and occupational sources.

Methods commonly utilized for the detection of heavy metals contaminants in food are the atomic absorption spectrophotometry (AAS) and neutron activation analysis (NAA). Neutron activation analysis is method of choice and considered more sensitive for arsenic, cadmium, mercury, and selenium; whereas AAS are preferred for lead and zinc. To determine methyl mercury, gas-liquid chromatographic (GLC) analysis is required.

ii. Control of Exposed Animal

Livestock should be quarantined whenever a severe heavy metal exposure occurs. It is recommended that cattle should not be slaughtered for at least 40-45 days after exposure to arsenic which results in clinical illness.

iii. Decontamination of Suspected Areas

Scientific methods should be applied to decontaminate water and sediments. Mercury polluted lakes and ponds should be prohibited for drinking for any animals and fishing as well.

iv. Removal of Toxicants from Food

Standard methods should be followed for removal of mercury and other heavy metals from milk, fish, and animal food products.

v. Removal of Hazards Container and Packaging Materials

Lead solder in food containers and lead colours in inks on printed plastic and paper container should be eliminated as soon as possible.

vi. Epidemiological Investigation

A thorough epidemiological study should be made for all outbreaks. This should enable one to determine the factors responsible for the intoxication so as to prevent future occurrences.

Toxicology of Metals

☆ *Naveen Kumar and Disha Pant*

Metal toxicosis in animals are often associated with industrial wastes (like mining operations, municipal sewage, power generation, coal burning) as well as commercial sources (like pesticides, medications, paint, and automotive products). Toxic metals may be cumulative and are stored in definite tissue locations inside body. Metals like lead accumulate in bone while arsenic accumulates in hair. These storage sites may serve as a reservoir for toxicants.

Special characteristic of heavy metals are environmentally stable, strong attraction to biological tissue and the slow elimination from biological system. Heavy metals exert their toxic effects by combining with one or more reactive group (ligand) essential for normal physiological function.

1. Arsenic

Arsenic is found in soil, water and air as a common environmental toxicant. It exists in several forms and has various uses, including insecticides, wood preservatives, herbicides, and even some medicinal uses. Arsenic constitutes one of the most important toxicological hazards to farm animals. Sometimes, arsenicals are added to the feed of poultry and animals to promote growth.

The arsenic atom exists in different forms like elemental, trivalent and pentavalent oxidation state. The toxicity of arsenicals varies with factors such as oxidation state of the arsenic, solubility, species of animal involved, duration of exposure, rate of its clearance from the body and its degree of accumulation in tissues. In general, toxicity increases in the sequence: organic arsenicals < arsenate (As^{5+}) < arsenite (As^{3+}) < arsine. The organic arsenicals usually are excreted more rapidly than are the inorganic forms.

Severe haemolysis is a unique characteristic of arsine poisoning and probably results from arsine (AsH_3; generated by electrolytic or metallic reduction of arsenic in nonferrous metal products) combining with haemoglobin and then reacting with oxygen to cause haemolysis. Haemolysis could be often rapid and fatal. The classic arsine triads are haemolysis, abdominal pain, and hematuria. Jaundice appears after 24 hours, if patient survives severe haemolysis, death often results from renal failure. Dimercaprol has no effect on the haemolysis, and no beneficial effects on renal function; thus it is not recommended.

Inorganic Arsenicals

Trivalent arsenicals are more soluble, therefore more toxic than pentavalent compounds. Pentavalent arsenicals have very low affinity for thiol-groups, and are much less toxic in contrast to the trivalent compounds. The lethal oral dose of sodium arsenite in most species is varies from 1-25 mg/kg. Cats may be more sensitive. Now a days poisoning is infrequent due to decreased use of these compounds as pesticides, baits, and wood preservatives. Lead arsenate (As^{5+}) is sometimes used as taenicide in sheep. Sometimes arsenite are also used as dips for tick control. Death of sheep may occur due to dipping in arsenical preparation.

Toxicokinetics

Soluble forms of arsenic compounds are well absorbed orally. Following absorption, most of the arsenic is bound to red blood cells (RBC) then distributed to several tissues such as in liver, kidney, heart, and lungs with highest concentration. In sub-chronic or chronic exposures, arsenic accumulates in skin, nails, hooves, and hair because of the high sulfhydryl content of keratin. Deposition in hair starts within 2 weeks after administration and arsenic stays fixed at this site for years. Arsenic readily crosses the placental barrier. The methylated forms of arsenic are less reactive with tissue constituents. The majority of the absorbed arsenic is excreted in the urine as inorganic arsenic or in methylated form. The half-life for the urinary excretion of arsenic is 3 to 5 days, which is shorter than other heavy metals.

Toxicodynamics

The mechanism of action of arsenic toxicosis varies with the type of arsenical compound. Tissues of gastro intestinal tract, liver, kidneys, lungs endothelium, and epidermis are considered more vulnerable to arsenic damage because they are rich in oxidative enzymes. Trivalent inorganic and aliphatic organic arsenic compounds exert their toxicity by interacting with sulfhydryl enzymes, resulting in disruption of cellular metabolism. Pentavalent arsenical is a known uncoupler of mitochondrial oxidative phosphorylation.

Clinical Findings

Poisoning due to arsenic is usually acute type with major effects on GIT and cardiovascular system.

In acute cases, capillary transudation of plasma produces vesicles under the GI mucosa, these eventually rupture, epithelial fragments slough off, and plasma is discharged into the lumen of intestine, where it coagulates and finally it is excreted through faeces as a mucosal shred. Tissue damage and the bulk cathartic action of the increased fluid in the lumen lead to increased peristalsis and characteristic watery diarrhoea ("rice-water stool"). Normal proliferation of epithelium is suppressed which accentuates the damage. Soon the faeces become bloody. Arsenic has a direct effect on the capillaries, causing damage to microvascular integrity, transudation of plasma, loss of blood, and hypovolemic shock. Profuse watery diarrhoea, sometimes tinged with blood, is characteristic, as are severe colic, dehydration, weakness, depression, weak pulse, and cardiovascular collapse. Other cardiovascular effects can result, including hypotension, congestive heart failure, and cardiac arrhythmias. The onset is rapid, and signs are usually seen within a few hours (or up to 24 hr). The course may run from hours to several weeks depending on the quantity ingested.

In per-acute poisoning, animals may simply be found dead. With chronic exposure to arsenic, gastrointestinal effects usually are not observed. Arsenic may cause severe renal damage. Initially the glomeruli are affected and oligourea, proteinuria and hematuria results. Skin is the major target organ of arsenic.

In chronic arsenic exposure, hyper pigmentation may be seen over the trunk and extremities. Commonly appears in finely freckled "raindrop pattern". Long-term ingestion of low doses of inorganic arsenical causes cutaneous vasodilatation. The most common early signs are muscle weakness and aching, skin pigmentation (especially of the neck, eyelids and nipples), hyperkeratosis and oedema. Dermatitis and keratosis of palms and soles are common features. Other sign and symptoms that should arouse suspicion of arsenic poisoning include garlic odour of the breath and perspiration, stomatitis, generalized itching and alopecia. Wasting, thirst, brick-red mucous membrane, normal temperature and weak irregular pulses are the characteristic lesion in chronic cases, but are very rarely observed.

Diagnosis

Chemical determination of arsenic in tissues (liver or kidney) or stomach contents provide confirmation. Toxicity is associated with a concentration >3 ppm arsenic (wet wt) of liver and kidneys. The determination of arsenic in stomach contents is of value usually within the first 24-48 hour after ingestion. The concentration of arsenic in urine can be high for several days after ingestion. Drinking water containing > 0.25 per cent arsenic is considered potentially toxic, especially for large animals.

Treatment

In animals with recent exposure, emesis should be induced (in capable species), followed by activated charcoal with a cathartic and then oral administration of GI protectants (in small animals, 1-2 hour after charcoal administration), such as kaolin-pectin, and fluid therapy as needed.In animals already showing clinical signs, aggressive fluid therapy and blood transfusion are suggested, if needed.

Chelation Therapy

- ☆ Often begun with dimercaprol (BAL; British antilewisite) @ 4-10 mg/kg, I/M, every 12 hours until recovery.
- ☆ The water soluble analogs of dimercaprol, DMPS (2, 3 dimercaptopropane -1- sulphonate) @ 100 mg/kg/day for 10-12 days and DMSA (dimercaptosuccinic acid or succimer)@ 30 mg/kg/day for 5-7 days are considered more effective than dimercaprol and could be given orally.

☆ d-Penicillamine may be substituted for dimercaprol;@ 10-50 mg/kg, orally, 3-4 times for 3-4 days. It has wide margin of safety.

In large animals, dimercaprol alone is not efficacious. Kidney and liver function should be monitored during treatment.

Organic Arsenicals

Some aliphatic arsenicals such as monosodium methanearsonate (MSMA) and disodium methanearsonate (DSMA) are occasionally used in agriculture as cotton defoliants and crabgrass killers.

Both compounds MSMA and DSMA persist in soil for longer period and their tendency to accumulate in plants creates poisoning in grazing animals. Phenylarsonic compounds are used as feed additives to improve production in swine and poultry rations. Toxicosis results from an excess of arsenic-containing additives in pig or poultry diets. Severity and rapidity of onset are dose-dependent. Signs may be delayed for weeks after incorporation of 2-3 times then the recommended level. It may occur within days when given > 10 times excess then the recommended levels.

Clinical signs, lesions, and treatment of organic arsenicals are similar to those of inorganic arsenicals. The earliest sign in pigs may be a reduction in weight gain, followed by incoordination, posterior paralysis, and eventually quadriplegia. Blindness is characteristic of arsanilic acid intoxication but not of other organic arsenicals. Once paralysis and blindness occurs, they are usually irreversible, but the animal remains alert and retains the appetite.

In ruminants, phenylarsonic toxicosis is similar to inorganic arsenic poisoning. Demyelination and gliosis of peripheral nerve, optic nerves and optic tract are usually seen in histopathology. In cattle, arsenic poisoning must be differentiated from lead poisoning, insecticide poisoning, and infectious diseases such as bovine viral diarrhoea.

There is no specific treatment, but the neurotoxic effects are usually reversible if the offending feed is withdrawn within 2-3 days of onset of ataxia.

2. Lead

Lead (Pb) is one of the most common causes of metallic poisoning in dog and cattle. It has worldwide distribution and accumulated in environment by industrial pollution. The primary environmental sources are leaded paint and drinking water. Vegetation grown in lead smelter areas where plants accumulate lead and contamination of vegetation on highways by exhaust fumes (petrol contains tetraethyl lead) are other important sources of lead poisoning. Feeding on crops sprayed with lead insecticides (lead arsenate) may also result in lead poisoning in animals. Lead has a profound effect on sulfhydryl containing enzymes, the thiol content of erythrocytes, antioxidant defences, and tissues rich in mitochondria which is reflected in the clinical syndrome.

Toxicokinetics

The major routes of absorption of lead are from the gastrointestinal tract and respiratory system. The degree of absorption and retention is influenced by dietary factors such as calcium or iron levels. Iron deficiency has been shown to enhance intestinal absorption of lead. Once lead is absorbed about 90 per cent lead of blood stream binds to haemoglobin in erythrocytes. Inorganic lead is distributed initially in the soft tissues (particularly the tubular epithelium) of kidney and in the liver. In time, lead is redistributed and deposited in bone, teeth and hair. About 95 per cent of body burden of the metal eventually is found in bone and the bone is considered to be "sink of lead". Only small quantities of inorganic lead accumulate in the brain (in gray matter and the basal ganglia). Lead readily crosses the blood-brain barrier and the placental barrier. The half-life of lead in blood is 1 to 2 months, and a steady state is achieved in about six months.

Lead (Pb^{2+}) and calcium (Ca^{2+}) may compete for a common transport mechanism, because there is a reciprocal relationship in their absorption. Some other factors that affect the kinetic of lead are:

- ☆ High intake of phosphate favours storage of lead in skeletal and lower the lead concentration in soft tissues. Conversely, a low phosphate intake mobilizes lead in bone and elevates its content in soft tissues.
- ☆ Vitamin "D" tends to promote the deposition of lead in bone if a sufficient amount of phosphate is available.
- ☆ Parathyroid hormones mobilize lead from the skeleton into blood and increase the rate of excretion in urine.

Toxicodynamics

Lead inhibits heme formation at several points, by inhibition of δ-aminolevulinate (δ-ALA) dehydratase and ferrochelatase, which are sulfhydryl dependent enzymes. Lead poisoning is characterized by accumulation of protoporphyrin IX in red blood cell, δ-ALA in plasma, and by increased urinary excretion of δ-ALA. Anemia and basophilic stippling of erythrocytes is uncommon in organic lead poisoning. Basophilic stippling (aggregation of ribonucleic acid) occurs in erythrocytes. This is result from the inhibitory effect of lead on the enzyme pyrimidine-5' nucleotidase.

Clinical Findings

Acute Lead Poisoning

Acute lead poisoning is relatively infrequent and occurs from ingestion of acid-soluble lead or inhalation of lead vapours. GI abnormalities including anorexia, colic, emesis, and diarrhoea or constipation, may be seen in dogs. Nausea, vomition (vomitus may be milky or rice water appearance) and severe abdominal pain. Acute lead poisoning is more common in young animals. In cattle, signs appear within 24-48 hour of exposure and include ataxia, blindness, jaw champing, muscle tremors, convulsions, and spastic twitching of eyelids.

Chronic Lead Poisoning

In cattle, syndrome may be divided into different categories: gastrointestinal, neuromuscular, haematological, renal and central nervous system (CNS). They may occur separately or in combination. Plumbism is seen in human. The nervous syndrome usually is more common in young one, whereas the gastrointestinal syndrome is more prevalent in adults. Neuromuscular effects include muscle weakness and easy fatigue that occurs long before actual paralysis. There usually is no sensory involvement.

CNS syndrome is termed as lead encephalopathy. There may increase in intracranial pressure. Other symptoms like anxiety, hysterical barking, jaw champing, salivation, blindness, ataxia, muscle spasms, opisthotonos and convulsions may develop. CNS depression rather than CNS excitation may be evident in some dogs. In horses, chronic syndrome is characterized by weight loss, depression, colic, diarrhoea, laryngeal or pharyngeal paralysis (roaring), and dysphagia that frequently tend to aspiration pneumonia. In avian species, anorexia, ataxia, loss of condition and anemia may notice.

Diagnosis

Physical examination does not easily distinguish lead colic from other abdominal disorders. Clinical suspicion should be confirmed by determination of the lead concentration in blood and protoporphyrin in erythrocytes. Haematological defects appear when blood concentration is near 80µg/dl or greater. Lead encephalopathy is usually apparent when lead concentration is > 100µg/dl. Hematologic abnormality may be indicative but not confirmatory of poisoning. Blood or urinary δ-aminolevulinic acid (δ-ALA) and free erythrocyte protoporphyrin levels are sensitive indicators of lead exposure but not a reliable indicator of lead poisoning. The common haematological finding of chronic lead intoxication is a hypochromic microcytic anemia and is morphologically similar to that resulting from iron deficiency. It could be due to decreased life span of the erythrocytes and an inhibition of heme synthesis. X-rays may show heavy, multiple bands of increased density in the growing long bones. The elevated concentrations of lead may be a cause of CNS and behavioural abnormalities.

Renal toxicity (interstitial nephropathy) is commonly observed in long term industrial lead exposure. Clinically, a Fanconi-like syndrome is seen with proteinuria, hematuria, and casts in the urine. Histologically, lead nephropathy is characterised by nuclear inclusion body, this appears early and can be resolves after chelation therapy.

Differential Diagnosis

Lead poisoning may be confused with other diseases that cause nervous or GI abnormalities. In cattle, such diseases may include polioencephalomalacia, nervous coccidiosis, tetanus, hypovitaminosis-A, hypomagnesemic tetany, nervous acetonemia, arsenic or mercury poisoning, brain abscess or neoplasia, rabies, listeriosis, and haemophilus infections. In dogs, rabies, distemper, and hepatitis may appear similar to lead poisoning.

Treatment

I. Supportive Treatment

☆ Seizures are treated with diazepam.

☆ Cerebral edema is treated with mannitol and dexamethasone.

☆ Fluid and electrolyte balance must be maintained.

☆ Cathartics such as magnesium sulphate (400 mg/kg, P.O.) or a rumenotomy may be useful to remove lead from the GI tract.

II. Chelation Therapy

Chelation therapy is indicated when blood lead concentration is high. Four chelators are generally employed; $CaNa_2$ EDTA (edetate calcium disodium), BAL/ dimercaprol (British Anti Lewisite), d-Penicillamine, and Succimer (meso 2,3-dimercaptosuccinic acid; DMSA).

☆ In large animals, calcium disodium edentate (Ca-EDTA) may be given IV or SC (110 mg/kg/day) for three days. This treatment should be repeated two days later.

In dogs, similar treatments per day may be administered in 5 per cent dextrose for 2-4 days. If clinical signs persist, an additional five day treatment may be given. Thiamine (2-4 mg/kg/day S.C.) reduce clinical manifestations and reduces tissue deposition of lead. Combined Ca-EDTA and thiamine produce most beneficial response.

☆ d-Penicillamine can be administered to dogs (@ 100-120 mg/kg/day, PO) for two week. However, undesirable side effects such as emesis and anorexia have been associated with this treatment. d-Penicillamine is not recommended for livestock.

☆ Succimer (meso 2,3-dimercaptosuccinic acid, DMSA) is a chelating agent that has proven to be effective in dogs (10-15 mg/kg, PO, t.i.d for 7 to 10 days) and is also useful in birds.

3. Mercury

Mercury (Hg) poisoning is common in both human and animal populations. Fossil fuels are an important environmental source of mercury poisoning. Commercial fish products have been associated with chronic mercury poisoning. Mercury is an important constituent of many drugs including antiseptics (*e.g.*, mercurochrome), antibacterial, diuretics, fungicides, skin ointment and laxative. In the environment, inorganic forms of mercury are converted to methylmercury under anaerobic conditions in the sediment of water. Similar conversions may also occur in the body. However, there is possibility of exposure to environmental sources of organic methylmercury.

Inorganic Mercury

Ingested inorganic mercury is poorly absorbed thus produces less toxic effects. These include the volatile elemental form of mercury (used in thermometers) and the salted forms mercuric chloride (sublimate) and mercurous chloride (calomel). Inorganic mercury are corrosive in nature, in large amount, may produce vomiting, diarrhoea and colic. Renal damage also occurs, with polydipsia and anuria in severe cases. Mercury vapour from elemental mercury produces corrosive bronchitis and interstitial pneumonia and, if not fatal, may lead to neurologic signs as do organic forms. Emesis followed by initiation of chelation therapy is recommended after acute oral ingestion.

Organic Mercury

Aryl mercurials (*e.g.* phenyl mercury, a fungicide) compounds are less prone to bioaccumulation. Animals poisoned by organic mercury exhibit stimulation of central nervous system and locomotor abnormalities. If cat is exclusively depends on commercial food there may be a chance of several neurological disturbances.

Minimata disease was an important outbreak of mercury poisoning that occurred due to methylmercur. Minimata is a small town of Japan, and its major industry empties their effluent directly into minimata Bay. Microorganism converts inorganic mercury to methylmercury in the rivers, lakes, and seas then this compound is taken up rapidly by plankton algae and is concentrated in fish via food chain. Residents of Minimata who consumed fish as a large proportion of their diet were the first to be poisoned.

Toxicokinetics

Insoluble inorganic mercurial compounds, such as calomel (Hg_2Cl_2), may undergo some oxidation to become soluble compounds that are more readily absorbed. Highest concentration of mercury is found in the kidneys, where they are retained for longer time than any other tissues. Inorganic mercurials do not readily pass through the blood-brain barrier and the placenta. The metal is excreted in the urine and faeces. Elemental mercury is not toxic when ingested because of very low absorption form gastric tract. Mercury vapour is completely absorbed by the lungs and crosses membrane more readily than the divalent mercury. A significant amount of the vapour enters the brain before it is oxidized to divalent mercuric cations (Hg^{2+}) by catalase in the erythrocytes. Central nervous system toxicity is thus more prominent after exposure to mercury vapour than to divalent forms of the metal.

The organic mercurials absorbed via all routes bioaccumulate in the brain and to some extent in the kidneys and muscle. The organic mercurials cross the blood-brain-barrier and the placenta barrier, and produce neurological and teratogenic effects more than that to inorganic mercury salts. Organic mercurials are more uniformly distributed to the various tissues than the inorganic salts. A significant portion of the body burden of organic mercurials is in the red blood cells. Mercury concentrates in hair because of its high sulfhydryl content. Excretion of methyl mercury is mainly through faeces in the form of conjugates with glutathione. The half-life of different form of mercurial compounds in blood is between 45 to 90 days.

Toxicodynamics

Like inorganic arsenicals, mercury readily forms covalent bonds with sulphur, and this property accounts for most of the toxic effect of metal. Even in low concentration, mercurial are capable of inactivating sulfhydryl enzymes and interfering cellular function. Affinity of mercury for thiol provides the basis for treatment of mercury poisoning with agents such as dimercaprol and *d*-penicillamine.

Clinical Signs

All three forms of mercury (*i.e.* elemental, inorganic and organic forms) exhibit neurotoxicity, nephrotoxicity, and gastrointestinal (with ulceration and haemorrhage) toxicity. Mercury is also a mutagenic, teratogenic, carcinogenic, and embryocidal compound.

Inorganic salts of mercury (*e.g.* mercuric chloride) can produce severe acute toxicity. Inorganic mercury compounds largely accumulate in kidneys, and may damage them. Upon oral ingestion, they produce local corrosive effects on the gastrointestinal mucosa resulting into vomition, diarrhoea and severe haematochezia (fresh blood in stool), with evidence of mucosal sloughing in the stool, leading to shock (hypovolemic) and death.

Elemental (vapour) mercury is poorly absorbed from gastrointestinal tract. The primary target organs of elemental mercury are the brain and kidneys. Elemental mercury is lipid soluble and can cross the blood-brain barrier, while inorganic mercury compounds are lipid insoluble, rendering them unable to cross the blood-brain barrier. Acute exposure to high levels of mercury vapor can lead to severe lung damage (interstitial pneumonitis), even death due to hypoxia. Acute poisoning usually occurs accidently in industrial areas that are exposed to high levels of mercury vapor. Mercury vapor may also enter the brain through nasal cavity can produce central nervous system toxicity, which are commonly reversible.

Organic mercurial (methyl mercury) exposure mainly produces neurological symptoms which consist of visual disturbance, ataxia, paresthesis, hearing loss, mental deterioration, muscle tremor, paralysis and death. Mental retardation and some neuromuscular deficit may be observed in fetus.

Systemic toxicity may begin within a few hours after exposure and can last for several days. A strong metallic taste is followed by stomatitis with gingival irritation, breath, and loosening of the teeth. The most serious and frequently encountered systemic effect of inorganic mercury is renal toxicity. Acrodynia (pink disease), an allergic reaction commonly follows chronic exposure of inorganic mercury ions which is characterized by erythema of the extremities, photophobia, diaphoresis, anorexia, tachycardia, and either constipation or diarrhoea. Cats may show hind leg rigidity, cerebellar dysfunction, ataxia, and tremors.

Diagnosis

A history of exposure to mercury is valuable for diagnosis of mercury poisoning. Clinical suspicions can be confirmed by laboratory analysis. The blood mercury is a useful biomarker after short term and high level exposure, whereas the urine mercury is the ideal biomarker for long term exposure to both elemental and inorganic mercury. In contrast, excretion of mercury in urine is a poor indicator of the amount of methyl mercury in the blood, because it is eliminated mainly in faeces.

Hair is rich in sulfhydryl groups, and the concentration of mercury in hair is about 250-300 times than in blood. Histological lesions include degeneration of neurons and perivascular cuffing in the cerebrocortical gray matter, cerebellar atrophy of the granular layer, and damage to Purkinje cells.

Differential Diagnosis

Conditions like tremor and ataxia must be differentiated from the symptom of other metals, insecticides, and cerebellar lesions due to feline parvovirus. Laboratory diagnosis should be differentiated between normal concentrations of mercury (especially whole blood, kidney, and brain) and concentrations associated with poisoning in tissue.

Treatment

Emesis can be induced if the patient is conscious and alert. Activated charcoal may be recommended. Neurologic signs may be irreversible once they develop. Mercury excretion can be increased by using chelating agents, such as dimercaprol (or British anti-lewisite), penicillamine and 2,3-dimercapto-1-propanesulfonic acid(Succimer).The short chain organic mercurial (especially methyl mercury) are the most difficult forms of mercury to mobilize from the body, probably due to their poor reactivity with chelating agents.

- ☆ Dimercaprol: At the dose of 3 mg/kg body wt, IM, every 4 hr for the first 2 days, q.i.d on the third day, and b.i.d until the complete recovery.
- ☆ Succimer: It is water soluble and less toxic dimercaprol; is a chelator of choice for organic mercury poisoning.
- ☆ Penicillamine: Dose rate of 15-50 mg/kg, PO, may be used only after the gut is free of ingested mercury.

Use of polythiol resin has advantage over penicillamine. It does not cause redistribution of mercury in the body.

☆ Haemodialysis has very little advantage in the treatment of poisoning because methylmercury concentrates in erythrocytes and very little amount is present in the plasma.

4. Selenium

Common sources of selenium poisoning are plants. Plants containing high selenium concentrations are the most important source of acute selenium poisoning in cattle, sheep and horses. Other sources are medicated shampoo, lubricating oils, fungicides and insect repellents.

It is an essential element, often used as micronutrient in diet to prevent several deficiency diseases such as white muscle disease in cattle and sheep, hepatosis dietetica in pigs, and exudative diathesis in chickens. All animal species are susceptible to selenium toxicosis and it is more common in forage eating animals when dietary selenium level exceeds 5 ppm.

Toxicokinetics

Selenium is readily absorbed from gut and distributed throughout the body, particularly in liver, kidneys and spleen. After absorption of organic selenium (selanomethionine), a selenide form is oxidized into salenite which is responsible for toxicosis. In general, a single oral dose of selenium *i.e.* 1-5 mg/kg body weight is lethal to most animals. Chronic toxicosis with organic selenium concentration of 10 to 40 mg/kg in different species has been reported. Chronic exposure results in large concentration in hair and hoof of affected animals. Gastrointestinal signs and lesions in acute selenium toxicity are due to the irritant nature of selenium in large concentration.

Toxicodynamics

Selenium is a component of the glutathione peroxidase enzyme that acts as an antioxidant. Most effects of selenium toxicity are due to the direct inhibition of cellular oxidation/reduction reactions, and the replacement of sulphur in the body. Altered sulphur containing amino acids affects cell division and growth; especially the cells that form keratin and sulphur-containing keratin are susceptible. Therefore, selenium poisoning weakens the hooves and hair, which tends to fracture.

Clinical Signs

Main classical sign is greying of dark hair coat. Other signs are diarrhoea, anemia, alopecia, rough dull hair, ataxia, stiffness, paralysis of limb, cracking of hooves and focal symmetric polioencephalomalacia.

Three classical syndromes of selenium poisoning are observed in animals, one acute and two chronic forms (*i.e.* blind staggers and alkali disease).

(A) Acute Toxicosis

Acute intoxication is very rare, can occur in animals as a result of consumption of highly seleniferous forage or grains. Young animals are most susceptible to acute parenteral selenium toxicosis. Cattle ingested selenium in feed @ 10 to 25 mg/ kg body weight are prone to acute poisoning. Clinical signs are characterized by abnormal behaviour, respiratory difficulty, gastrointestinal upset, and sudden death. Abnormal posture and depression, anorexia, unsteady gait (peculiar "rooted-to-one spot" with lowered head), diarrhoea, colic, increased pulse and respiration rates, frothy nasal discharge, moist rales, cyanosis and death may occur due to respiratory arrest. Sheep may die suddenly without showing any clinical sign of toxicity.

(B) Chronic Toxicosis

Chronic selenium poisoning usually develops when livestock consume seleniferous feed or fodder containing 5 to 50 mg of selenium for many weeks or months. Naturally occurring seleno amino acids in plants are readily absorbed. Two types of chronic selenium poisoning have been observed in animals: blind staggers and alkali disease

Blind staggers is no longer believed to be caused by selenium but by sulphate toxicity due to consumption of high sulfate containing alkali water. Excess sulfate (> 2 per cent of diet) leads to polioencephalomalacia, a classical lesion of blind staggers). Animal affected by blind staggers show symptoms like drooling of saliva, pale mucosa, grinding of teeth, walking in circle, corneal opacity, generalized muscle paralysis (including muscles of tongue and swallowing) and animal dies from respiratory failure.

Alkali disease is characterized by cracking of hooves at the coronary band, lameness, and loss of hair usually at the tip of tail. Deformed hooves may appear 15-18 cm long and turned upward. In sows, conception rate decreases and mortality of piglets at birth increases. Egg with >2.5 ppm of selenium level have low hatchability and embryos are usually deformed, without beaks and with ropy feathers. Biochemical changes in blood include decreased fibrinogen levels and prothrombin activity, increased serum alkaline phosphates, ALT, AST and succinic dehydrogenase activity.

Post Mortem Lesions

Ascites is a common finding. Animal die of acute toxicosis shows pulmonary congestion and oedema, degenerative changes in liver and kidneys. In blind staggers, necrosis and cirrhosis of liver, enlargement with localised haemorrhagic areas on spleen, congestion of renal medulla, epicardial petechial hyperamia and ulceration of abdomen and small intestine, erosion of articular surface (particularly of tibia) are seen at necropsy. In alkali disease lesions almost resemble those of blind stagger.

Diagnosis

Diagnosis is based on history, clinical signs, necropsy findings and laboratory confirmation of selenium level in diet, blood and tissue samples. Selenium levels beyond 5 ppm in diet are indicative of selenium toxicity.

Differential Diagnosis

Conditions that mimic the chronic selenosis (alkali disease) include ergotism, molybdenosis, perosis, laminitis and polioencephalomalacia (metabolic neuromuscular disorder of goat) due to thiamine deficiency. The odour of rotten garlic in a fresh carcass is suggestive of acute toxicosis but absence of such an odour may not completely rule out this condition because the volatile selenide may escape quickly.

Treatment

There is no specific treatment or antidote for selenium toxicosis.

5. Copper

Almost all species are susceptible to copper poisoning but sheep are most frequently affected. Dog breed Bedlington terrier has an inherited sensitivity to copper toxicosis. Copper play vital role in physiological system of animal body. Low levels of molybdenum or sulphate promote copper toxicosis. There is variation in susceptibility to copper poisoning among species. Equine have less susceptibility and can tolerate high concentrations of copper in the diet.

Copper poisoning occurs in animals when grazing immediately after fertilization, pastures grown on soils containing high concentrations of copper, pastures treated with antifungal drugs containing copper, administration of mineral mix with excessive copper concentration. The stressed animal has an increased susceptibility to copper poisoning because the stress promotes release of copper accumulated in the liver into bloodstream.

Toxicokinetics

Administration of selenium reduces biliary excretion of copper resulting in accumulation of copper in hepatocyte exposing the animals to a chronic copper poisoning. The large concentration of copper in the cells causes inhibition of essential metabolic enzymes that may lead to liver dysfunction. Damaged liver releases large amount of copper into blood circulation. The copper enter in erythrocytes and is excreted within 24 hours in urine before the onset of haemolytic crisis. The hemolytic crisis may be precipitated by many factors including transportation, pregnancy, lactation, strenuous exercise and unbalanced nutrition.

Toxicodynamics

In the erythrocytes, haemoglobin (Hb) is converted to methaemoglobin (met-Hb) by cupric ion (Cu^{2+}), simultaneously reduction in glutathione (GSH) concentration in the erythrocytes. This is due to monovalent copper is produced following the reduction of divalent copper during the conversion of Hb to met-Hb. The reduction in concentration of glutathione makes erythrocyte very fragile that leads to sudden and massive lysis of erythrocytes *i.e.* haemolytic crisis. Just before the onset of haemolytic crisis there is marked increase in packed cell volume (PCV) and also increase in the number and size of erythrocytes. Cytoplasmic inclusion appears in the renal tubules. As consequences of haemolytic crisis, there is failure of kidneys and elevation of plasma creatinine phosphokinase (CPK) concentration indicating damage to skeletal muscles. The animal that survive haemolytic crisis may die due to uraemia. Sheep died of copper poisoning may show lesion in the brain.

Clinical Signs

Acute Copper Poisoning

Acute poisoning occurs when animal gets access to feed contaminated with copper salts. Some copper containing drugs are used for treatment of disease that may cause severe fatalities even at the recommended dose level. Copper edetate used in the treatment of swayback disease in lambs has been reported to cause fatalities. Losses in lambs occur after treatment of foot-rot disease, either due to contamination of ewe udder or from drinking of foot-rot bath water.

Acute poisoning causes severe gastroenteritis characterized by abdominal pain diarrhoea, anorexia, dehydration and shock. Faeces of affected animals are deep green in colour due to the presence of copper-chlorophyll compounds. Haemolysis and hemoglobinuria may develop after 2-3 days, if the animal survives the gastro intestinal disturbances.

Chronic Copper Poisoning

A high copper: molybdenum ratio within plants can cause chronic copper poisoning since low molybdenum intake enhances storage of copper in the liver. Chronic poisoning is seen most commonly in sheep when ingested excessive amounts of copper over a prolonged period. Damage of liver by grazing of plants like *Hellotroplumeuropeum* can lead to excessive accumulation of copper causing hepatogenous chronic copper poisoning raising the risk of haemolytic crisis. Such plant contains hepatotoxic alkaloids that result in retention of excessive copper in the liver. Sudden increase in blood copper concentrations causes lipid peroxidation and intravascular hemolysis. Severe hepatic insufficiency is responsible for deaths. Chronic copper poisoning takes places in three stages:

Stages	Duration	Clinical Signs
First stage	last for 2-3 months -	No clinical signs observed
Second stage	last for 14-25 days -	Impairment of liver function
Third stage	lasting for 2-5 days -	Haemolytic crisis, generalised icterus, haemoglobinuria and recumbence

Post Mortem Lesions

In acute cases severe gastroenteritis with erosions and ulceration in the abomasum of ruminants are observed. Blood is found coagulated at the time of death.

In Chronic cases, swollen gunmetal coloured kidneys (showing haemorrgagic mettling when capsule is removed), port-wine coloured urine, enlarged spleen with brown-black (blackberry jam) parenchyma, enlarged liver (yellow in colour and friable) and generalised icterus are observed. Histologically, centrilobular hepatic and renal tubular necrosis are noticed.

Diagnosis

Blood copper concentrations are increased often exceeding to 15-20 µg/ml than the normal level. Evidence of blue-green ingesta and deep green coloured feces are there.

Differential Diagnosis

Copper poisoning must be differentiated from that mimic the haemolytic conditions such as leptospirosis, anaplasmosis and bacillary hemoglobinuria. The levels of copper in tissues must be determined to rule out other causes of haemolytic disease.

Treatment

Symptomatic treatment may be useful in acute toxicity. Dietary supplementation with zinc acetate may be useful to reduce the absorption of copper.

6. Molybdenum

Ruminants are more susceptible to molybdenum toxicity than non-ruminant animals. Cattle are less tolerant than sheep. The sources of poisoning are high concentration of molybdenum in plants, copper deficient plants, paint factory, oil refineries and application of fertilizer containing molybdenum. Susceptibility of ruminants to molybdenum toxicity depends on a several factors. Animals ingest feed with high concentration of molybdenum or when feed has deficiency of copper. Tolerance to molybdenum toxicity decreases as the intake of copper decreases.

Toxicokinetics

Molybdenum compounds are both rapidly absorbed and rapidly excreted. The storage is occurs throughout the body tissues, but found highest concentration in kidneys and bones. The retention and excretion is considerably affected by the amount of copper and inorganic sulphate in the diet.

The metabolism of copper, molybdenum, and inorganic sulfate have complex inter relationship. Increasing inorganic sulphate intake promotes the excretion of large quantities of molybdenum in urine. Low dietary sulphate causes high blood molybdenum levels due to decreased excretion.

Toxicodynamics

Molybdenum is an essential component of metalloenzymes (xanthine oxidase and aldehyde oxidase) that are necessary for maintaining health of animal. In feed of cattle, copper: molybdenum ratio of 6:1 is considered ideal; 3:1 is border line and less than 2:1 is toxic. In Rumen, interaction of molybdates and sulfides gives rise to mono, di, tri and tetra thiomolybdates. Copper reacts with tetrathiomolybdates in the rumen to form an insoluble complex that is poorly absorbed in gastrointestinal tract. On this basis tetrathiomolybdate is used in treating and preventing copper toxicity in sheep.

Clinical Signs

Clinical sign of molybdenum toxicity in cattle appears within 10 to 15 days of grazing on affected pastures, characterized by persistent and severe scouring with liquid faeces full of gas bubbles (peat scour or teart), anorexia, immune suppression and dudley hair (especially around eyes which gives a "spectacled appearance"). The affected animals show abnormal pacing gait (*i.e.,* pacing diseases). Sheep, and young animals in particular show stiffness of back and legs with reluctant to rise, which is known as enzootic ataxia or swayback diseases. Lambs are severely incoordinated gait, ataxic and blind. Sheep develop pica. Relatively low levels of molybdenum may exert direct effects on reproduction that is independent of alterations in copper metabolism.

Other signs of toxicity include unthriftiness, anemia (hypochromic type), emaciation, joint pain (lameness), osteoporosis and decreased fertility. Anemia is mainly due to copper deficiency occurring as a result of reduction in activity of sulphide oxidase in the liver.

Differential Diagnosis

Molybdenum poisoning must be differentiated from paratuberculosis and deficiency of copper.

Diagnosis

A tentative diagnosis can be made if diarrhoea stops within a few days of oral dosing with copper. Diagnosis can be confirmed by demonstrating abnormal concentration of molybdenum and low level of copper in feed and blood sample. The molybdenum is toxic to hepatocytes and renal tubular epithelial cells, producing periacinar to massive hepatic necrosis and nephrosis.

Treatment

Scouring can be controlled by daily administration of 5 mg of copper/kg of food.

7. Cadmium

Cadmium is nonessential element that accumulates in environment as a result of industrial exposure. Cadmium is widely used as a colouring pigment in paints, and in batteries. In nature, cadmium occurs in association with zinc and lead. Cadmium is a by-product of zinc and lead mining. Cereal grains (such as rice and wheat) and other pasture grasses concentrate cadmium when they are grown in soils with high concentrations of cadmium. Drinking water normally does not contribute significantly to cadmium intake. Shellfish, animal liver and kidney are among foods that can have concentrations of cadmium, even under normal conditions. The exact mechanism of cadmium toxicity is not well known but lipid peroxidation may be an early and sensitive consequence of cadmium toxicity.

In Fuchu, Japan, shortly after world war II, a large number of people complained of rheumatic and myalgic pains; the disease was named *itai-itai* (ouch-ouch). It was documented that cadmium had washed into the local rice fields from the effluent of a lead-zinc processing plant.

Toxicokinetics

Cadmium occurs only in divalent state (Cd^{2+}) and does not form other stable compound like alkyl or organometallic compounds. Cadmium is absorbed poorly from the gastrointestinal tract whereas absorption from the respiratory tract appears to be more complete. After absorption, cadmium is transported in blood, bound mainly to blood cells and albumin. Cadmium is distributed first to the liver and then is redistributed slowly to the kidney as cadmium-metallothionein (Cd-MT) complex. After distribution, approximately 50 per cent of total body burden is found in the liver and kidney. Metallothionein is low molecular weight protein with high affinity for metals such as cadmium and zinc. MT is inducible by exposure to several metals, including cadmium. Cadmium accumulates in the body because of its very slow urinary excretion. However, its biological half-life may be up to 10-40 years.

Diagnosis

Acute poisoning usually results from inhalation of cadmium dusts and fumes. In the case of oral intake, these include nausea, vomiting, salivation, diarrhoea, and abdominal cramps. The vomitus and diarrhoea are often bloody. Cadmium is more toxic when inhaled. The respiratory symptoms appear within few hours, includes irritation of respiratory tract, early pneumonitis and chest pains.

In chronic poisoning, cadmium binds to metallothionein, in which form it is stored. Some metallothionein bound cadmium leaks into plasma, and then reaches to kidney as inorganic cadmium. With more severe exposure of kidney, glomerular injury occurs, filtration is decreased and there is aminoaciduria, glycosuria, and proteinuria.

Excretion of β_2- microglobulin in urine appears to be a sensitive but not specific index of cadmium-induced nephrotoxicity. Retinol-binding protein may be a better marker, but its measurement is not generally available. Other symptoms of Cd toxicity include dyspnea, hypertension, osteomalacia and testicular necrosis.

Treatment

Effective therapy for cadmium poisoning is difficult and seldom achieved. Respiratory support and steroid therapy may be necessary. Some veterinarians recommend chelation therapy with $CaNa_2$ EDTA. The use of dimercaprol and substituted dithiocarbamates appears promising for individuals with chronic exposure to cadmium.

Toxicology of Non-Metals

☆ *Ratn Deep Singh and Hitesh B. Patel*

1. Phosphorus

In the body, about 80-85 per cent of phosphorus is present in inorganic or phosphate form (PO_4^{3-}), mainly in bones and teeth as crystalline hydroxyapatite, an essential ingredient, which is a mineral form of calcium and phosphorus. Rest 15-20 per cent of adult body phosphorus is found in the soft tissues. Inorganic phosphorus is required for biosynthesis of ATP, phospholipids, nucleic acids and enzyme co-factors. In nature, elemental phosphorus exists in two forms *viz.* yellow and red phosphorus. Red phosphorus is non-toxic whereas yellow phosphorus, also known as white phosphorus, is toxic. Yellow or white phosphorus is oil-soluble, waxy solid having garlic-like odour and ignites when exposed to the air, hence is stored under water. Industrial use of white phosphorus involves manufacturing of fertilizers, food additives, fireworks, pesticides and cleaning compounds.

Farm animals are rarely intoxicated by phosphorus. Horses, sheep and dogs are being reported to be affected by phosphorus toxicity. Toxic levels of phosphorus in animals greatly vary depending on the state of the phosphorus being ingested. In laboratory species, LD_{50} of different compounds of phosphorus ranges between 1.38 to 10.6 g per kg of body weight.

Sources of Poisoning

1. Earlier, white phosphorus was used in making rodenticide bait and thus, causing toxicity in pets due to accidental ingestion.

2. Feed having improper Ca:P ratio (less than 2:1). More use of diets which are rich in phosphorus and low in calcium, *e.g.* excessive wheat bran feeding in equines cause "Bran disease" and likewise organ meats in dogs cause hyperphosphatemia. Thus, phosphorus toxicities in animals are mainly associated with metabolic disorders of calcium as a result of diets high in phosphorus but low in calcium.

3. Accidental ingestion of phosphate based fertilizers.

Toxicokinetics

White phosphorus is highly lipid soluble agent which can be absorbed into the body by inhalation (it produces white smoke on air exposure), ingestion, or dermal exposures. Following fair and rapid absorption through intestine, phosphorus is oxidized into phosphates in circulation. It is primarily eliminated in urine and faces. As phosphates are readily excreted in urine, generally they are well tolerated. Some part is also excreted through pulmonary circulation and thus expired air may have characteristic garlic-like odour.

Toxicodynamics

Toxicity of phosphorus may occur in many ways and their mechanisms are as follows:

1. White phosphorus act as strong irritant and corrosive to gastro-intestinal mucosa and exerts necrotizing effect.

2. Compounds of phosphorus in excess act as protoplasmic poison and have direct cardiotoxic effect.

3. Phosphates in excess cause hepatic and renal degenerations.

4. They induce formation of phosphate based urinary calculi.

5. High dietary phosphorus or phosphates leads to decreased absorption of calcium and decreased plasma calcium which causes nutritional secondary hyperthyroidism particularly in horses. There is more stimulated secretion of parathyroid hormone (PTH) and thus, more bone mineral reabsorption. When these demineralized bones are replaced by fibrous connective tissues, it leads to enlargement of bones known as fibrous osteodystrophy. In equines, the condition of enlarged facial bones due to phosphorus toxicity is known as 'Big-Head Disease'.

Clinical Signs

☆ Abdominal pain (colic) and severe diarrhea due to gastro-intestinal irritation, there is profuse vomiting in able species. Hematemesis is commonly observed.

☆ There may be painful muscular spasms and tremors due to low level of plasma calcium.

☆ Hepatic failure and jaundice is observed in serious cases.

☆ Urolithiasis (urinary calculi) may be seen characterized by progressive oliguria and anuria. Calculi problem due to phosphorus toxicity are more observed in male sheep.

☆ Rarely, neurological disorders and paralysis are observed.

☆ Dermal exposure of white phosphorus causes second to third degree burns on the skin, having a characteristic yellow color and garlic-like odour.

☆ Long-term or chronic exposure to white phosphorus in humans causes necrosis of the jaw, known as "Phossy Jaw".

Post-mortem Findings

Common P.M. findings for phosphorus toxicity in animals include severe gastro-enteritis, fatty degenerations of liver, muscles and blood vessel endothelium, and disfigurement of bones.

Diagnosis

Diagnosis of phosphorus toxicity is based on history, clinical signs and P.M. lesions described above and plasma phosphorus levels. There will be elevated hepatic enzymes (ALT, AST) and bilirubin levels. A garlic-like odour comes from breath or vomitus of affected animals which may illuminate in dark.Range of normal plasma phosphorus level in adult horse and dog is 1.9 to 5.4 and 2.5 to 6.0 mg/dL, respectively. Differential diagnosis should be considered with other inorganic elements (As, Hg, Pb) and organophosphorus compounds. Hyperphosphatemia in dogs is also seen in conditions *viz.* bone-cancer, osteoporosis, leptospirosis and thyroid disorders.

Treatment

There is no specific antidote available and prognosis is guarded to grave for phosphorus toxicity. Effort to treatment is only based on symptomatic and supportive therapy. Absorbent like activated charcoal is effective. Use of emetics can be attempted in acute cases. Use of demulcent and astringents are beneficial. Electrolytes should be provided. Purgatives may be indicated but never use oily purgatives as they favour absorption of phosphorus. Copper sulphate is good *in vitro* neutralizer of phosphorus and may be cautiously used in dermal burns as copper is readily absorbed from such burns. Tap water irrigation is also useful in dermal burns.

2. Nitrate and Nitrite

Nitrate (NO^{3-}) compounds are practically non-toxic or lesser toxic in nature and their toxic symptoms are mainly related to gastro-intestinal system, whereas nitrite (NO^{2-}) compounds are far more toxic *i.e.* about 6-10 times more than nitrate (NO^{3-}) compounds and mainly affect the haemoglobin. Both compounds are water soluble and hence water contaminated with these compounds can cause toxicity. Water sourced from well may contain high nitrate concentrations due to runoff from the use of nitrogen-containing agricultural fertilizers and seepage of organic nitrogen-containing materials from animal wastes or septic sewer systems. In domestic ruminants, forage rich in nitrates are main source of poisoning and are not uncommon events. In plants, soil nitrogen is fixed by nitrogen fixing bacteria through root nodules and then after ammonification and nitrification first converted into nitrites and then in nitrates which is mainly stored in stem and stalks and further utilized for amino-acid synthesis.

The order of species susceptibility to nitrate and nitrite poisoning is Pig > Cattle > Sheep > Goats > Horse. Pigs are the most susceptible species for nitrate poisonings but occurrence is less reported.

- ☆ In general, ruminants are more susceptible to nitrate poisoning than non-ruminants because nitrate in forage is converted into nitrite in the rumen by rumen microbes.

- ☆ Goats are less susceptible because they have habit of selective leaf grazing and leaves are having low content of nitrates than in stem or stalks.

- ☆ In horses, nitrate is converted to nitrite in large intestine, closer to the end of the digestive tract, where there is less opportunity for the nitrite to be absorbed by blood and thus considered less susceptible to toxicity.

- ☆ Human infants less than six month of age are the most susceptible group to methemoglobinemia caused by nitrate poisoning and the condition is known as 'blue-baby syndrome'.

Sources of Poisoning

Forage Plants

In animals, nitrate rich forage plants are main source of poisoning for nitrate and nitrite toxicity. In stress conditions, nitrogen metabolism of plants gets disturbed and accumulation of nitrate is increased. This increase is seen more in some plants known as nitrate-accumulator plants, *e.g.* maize (*Zea mays*), lucerne (alfalfa), oat (*Avena sativa*), sugar-beet, turnip, berseem (*Trifoliumal exandrinum*), bajra (*Pennisetum glaucum*), *etc.* Some cyanogenic plants like sorghum (*Sorghum vulgare*) and sudan grass are also known to be nitrate rich plants. Some weeds like *Kochia* and wild sun-flower accumulates more nitrate than the crops or forage grasses. For cattle, fodder or forage containing more than 5000 ppm nitrate have potential to cause toxicity. Following are the factors which may contribute to increased nitrate levels in plants or their toxicity level in animals:

a) Fodders grown under climatic stress like frost or chilling weather and drought

b) Lack of sun-light or plants grown in shaded area

c) Plant diseases like wilting

d) Application of herbicides like 2,4 – D (2,4-Dichlorophenoxyacetic acid)

e) Use of nitrogen based fertilizers

f) High use of monensin as a feed additive, as it changes rumen environment and favours growth of micro-organisms leading to more conversion of nitrate into nitrites

g) Higher in younger plants

h) More in bottom of stem or stalk

i) Soil deficient in Sulphur (S) and Molybdenum (Mo)

j) Ingestion of urine or faeces mutilated fodder

Hay and Silage

Hays are rich in preformed nitrites, hence are more toxic, whereas silage have 30-60 per cent low nitrates than the untreated forage due to fermentation. Since during the process of silage-making there is emission of nitrogen dioxide (NO_2) gas, there is chance of occupational hazard for the workers or labours involved in the silo filling process. This toxicity of NO_2 gas is also known as 'Silage gas poisoning' or 'Silo's filler disease'.

Drinking Water

If contaminated with fertilizers, animal waste or decaying organic matters or if water source is from an area where soil is rich in nitrates may cause toxicity. High environmental ammonia too can condense in the water form and may increase the level. Water containing more than 1000 ppm poses risk of toxicity in livestock. Algal bloom or algae growth in water source reduces its nitrate content whereas coli form bacterial growth increases the nitrate level of water.

i. Accidental poisoning: Due to ingestion of nitrate salt containing fertilizers or chemicals like potassium nitrate.

ii. Treatment of animals with sodium nitrite in the cases misdiagnosed as cyanide toxicity.

Toxicokinetics

After absorption nitrate is reduced into nitrite by microbial reductases in ruminants. This nitrite is utilized by rumen microbes and converted into ammonia as a nitrogenous source. However, excessive nitrite gets accumulated in rumen, from where it is readily absorbed into blood stream. In monogastric animals, nitrate is rapidly and almost completely absorbed in the proximal small intestine. Nitrates and nitrites are distributed widely through the circulation. Excretion is done mainly through urine but salivary excretion also occurs. Hence, salivary, plasma, and urinary levels of nitrate and then nitrite rise abruptly after ingestion of nitrates.

Toxicodynamics

Nitrate ions in excess cause irritation to the gastrointestinal mucosa. In blood, nitrite ion is exchanged with chloride ion to enter the RBCs. Nitrite ions produce toxicity mainly by conversion of haemoglobin (Hb) into methaemoglobin (MetHb),and also cause peripheral vasodilatation and hypotension due to relaxation of vascular smooth muscles resulting into further failure of circulation. Normal haemoglobin contains iron into ferrous state (Fe^{2+}) whereas methaemoglobin is oxidized form of haemoglobin which contains iron in ferric state (Fe^{3+}) with reduced affinity for molecular oxygen (O_2). Thus methaemoglobin does not accept or carry oxygen to various body tissues causing oxygen starvation to tissues. In body, RBC intrinsic reductase system gradually reduces MetHb into Hbwith the help of NADH dependent Diaphorase I and II enzymes. Clinical toxicity is observed when the conversion of Hb into MetHb exceeds 40 per cent in animals, whereas conversion more than 80 per cent is lethal. Magnitude of toxicity also depends upon the initial Hb level of the animal and hence in severe anemic animals, toxicity is seen even if conversion is about 20 per cent.

Clinical Signs

- ☆ Vomition (in able species), diarrhoea and colic due to nitrate ion effects on GI tract
- ☆ Difficulty in breathing (dyspnoea), rapid and noisy breathing with gasping
- ☆ Normal to sub-normal temperature, rapid but weak pulse and accelerated heart rate
- ☆ Cyanosis or blue-brownish discoloration of mucous membranes easily visible at conjunctiva, vulva and vagina and unpigmented areas of skin.
- ☆ Chocolate brown colour of the blood which does not change with time or after exposure to atmospheric oxygen.
- ☆ Abortion in pregnant animals.
- ☆ Salivation, bloat, staggering, muscular tremors, coma and death within 2-3 hours.
- ☆ Chronic nitrate toxicity is goitrogenic in sheep as it interferes with iodine metabolism.

Post-mortem Findings

There is severe reddening and stripping of stomach in monogastric animals whereas congestion, hyperaemia and oedema of ruminal, abomasal and intestinal mucosa in ruminants. Cyanotic carcass and dark coffee brown or chocolate colour blood is seen which is poorly clotted in dilated vessels. Pin point haemorrhages are present in internal organs like heart and lungs. Aborted fetuses may show ascites and hydrothorax.

Diagnosis

Based on history (nitrate content level of forage), clinical signs, post-mortem lesions described above, diphenylamine (DPA) test can be used as spot field test for detection of nitrates and nitrites. Formation of blue ring indicates positive result in DPA test. Readymade field kits based on diphenylamine reagent is also available in some countries. For analytical evidences, blood or ocular fluid level of nitrate and nitrites are useful indicators. Plasma is preferred over serum samples as nitrate is retained in the clot. Plasma or ocular nitrate level > 20 ppm and nitrite level > 0.5 ppm in such samples of ruminants suggests nitrate/nitrite toxicity. Differential diagnosis includes urea toxicity, grain overload, hypomagnesaemia and hypocalcaemia. Agents other than nitrate and nitrites, which may cause methaemoglobinaemia include chlorate, benzocaine, dapsone, sulfa drugs and acetaminophen in overdose.

Treatment

Methylene blue is an effective treatment for treating nitrate/nitrite poisoning which reduces methaemoglobin into haemoglobin using $NADPH_2$ reductase system of the body. This reduction yields free haemoglobin and forms leuco- methylene blue which further activates diaphorase I and II enzymes. Methylene blue is used as 1 per cent solution in normal saline and administered by slow IV route at the dose rate of 4.4- 8.8 mg/kg body weight in sheep and cattle, repeated at 4-6 hrs intervals initially. Treatment is given till the recovery is observed or given up to 5-7 days. However, in many countries, use of methylene blue in cattle is banned due to its longer residual problem in milk and meat. Supportive therapy like supplemental oxygen and symptomatic treatment are done as required. Vitamin C and chlortetracycline are proved as helpful aid in treatment. Chlortetracycline @ 2.2 mg/kg in feed may reduce extent of nitrate conversion into nitrites.

3. Common Salt

Common salt or sodium chloride (NaCl), popularly knowns as table salt, is essential in animals diet as it regulates osmotic balance of the body fluids especially extra-cellular fluid (ECF), maintains electrolyte balance, important for nerve impulse conduction, rhythmic maintenance of heart action and essential for diuresis mechanism. It also increases palatability of feed. Normally, blood contains 0.9 per cent NaCl. Both component of common salt is essential to body, as sodium ion (Na^+) is the major extracellular cation while chloride ion (Cl^-) is the major extracellular anion. Generally, it is required at the rate of 0.5-1 per cent in diet of animals and this requirement is higher in high lactating animals. Minor excess of sodium chloride in feed is well tolerated by animals if they have *ad libitum* access to drinking water. But restricted supply of drinking water to animals predisposes them to the salt-poisoning; hence the condition is also known as 'water-deprivation syndrome'. Animals can tolerate common salt at the rate up to 10 – 13 per cent in diet when water is freely available, but level of salt as low as 0.25 per cent in diet can cause toxicity if water is restricted. Since the sodium ions are responsible for the toxic response of common salt, this toxicity is also known as 'sodium-ion intoxication' and there is condition of hypernatremia in the body of affected animal. Oral LD_{50} of NaCl in rat and mouse is 3.0 and 4.0 g/kg body weight, respectively. Acute oral toxic dose for swine, cattle and horses is 2.2 g/kg body weight whereas for dog and sheep is 4.0 and 6.0 g/kg body weight, respectively. Thus, sheep is most resistant species to salt toxicity.

Swine and poultry are the two species most susceptible to salt poisoning. Order of susceptibility is Swine and Poultry > Cattle > Horse > Dogs > Sheep. Poultry are susceptible to common salt toxicity due to poor sense of taste, non-selective feeding behavior, low plasma protein and decreased glomerular filtration area.

Young animals and birds are more susceptible. Lactating dairy animals are relatively more susceptible than dry animals due to unstable fluid and electrolyte imbalance.

Sources of Poisoning

i. Accidental ingestion of salt or high consumption of salt rich diets (like salt-licks) causes salt-toxicity especially in water restricted animals. In cold countries, salt is used as de-icing agent on road which can be an exposure factor especially for birds.

ii. Salt hungry animals, to whom salt in diet is withhold for considerable period, can consume much salt if re-introduced in their diet.

iii. Use of ground water source, which are high in salt content, as drinking water for animals; or accidental consumption of sea-water by pets/livestock.

iv. Overdose of salt when used as emetics to induce vomition in small animals.

Toxicokinetics

Following ingestion, there is rapid absorption of sodium and chloride mainly from small intestine and about 85-95 per cent of NaCl is absorbed. Significant portion of absorbed sodium and chloride are recycled again into the intestinal tract via salivary, pancreatic, and intestinal epithelial secretions, as well as bile. High concentration of sodium ions in intestine is required for transportation of glucose, amino acids, and other nutrients across the mucosa. Excess sodium ions in blood diffuse into cerebrospinal fluid (CSF). Sodium is efficiently excreted via the kidney if water is sufficient in the body. Some excretion of salt occurs through skin (sweat) also.

Toxicodynamics

Toxic signs of salt poisoning are mainly due to cellular dehydration, tissue shrinking and oedema. Following mechanisms act together to produce toxic effects of sodium ion toxicity:

1. Increased blood sodium level or hypernatremia in reflex causes arousal of thirst and if water is not made available to animal, it will produce hypertonicity of blood which causes toxicity. It results into withdrawal of water from capillary vascular endothelial cells causing their shrinkage and increased permeability in important organs like brain, kidney and lungs. Thus, there is cerebral oedema, pulmonary oedema and shrinkage of renal tubular epithelium with deposition of sodium crystals in tubules.

2. Acute high doses of NaCl in gastro-intestinal lumen act as a saline purgative withdrawing the water resulting in diarrhea and animal becomes dehydrated.

3. Cerebrocortical damage and alteration in nerve conduction due to altered Na^+-K^+ pump leads to clinical signs due to effects on nervous system.

Clinical Signs

Swine

Loss of appetite, intense thirst, champing of jaws, frothing at the mouth, watery diarrhea, constipation, phases of convulsive seizures, stupor, hyperesthesia, pruritis, wandering and head-pressing, circling or pivoting around a limb, dog-sitting posture, comatose and death.

Poultry

Intense thirst, gasping (dyspnea), wet faeces (diarrhea), foaming from mouth or fluid discharge from beak, weakness, and paralysis of legs.

Cattle

Loss of condition due to anorexia, dehydration, ataxia (muscular weakness), muscular fasciculations and tremors, sometimes blindness, paddling, partial paralysis with knuckling at fetlock joint, dragging of hind limb while walking, and sternal or lateral recumbency.

Dogs

Vomition, profuse watery diarrhea, lethargy, ataxia, convulsions and coma, blindness in severe cases.

Post-mortem Findings

Congested and inflamed gastric mucosa with pin point ulcers and hemorrhages, cerebral and pulmonary oedema, hydropericardium, hepatic and renal congestions, and renal tubular damage in various species are noticed. Polioencephalomalacia in catlle and meningioencephalitis with eosinophilic perivascular cuffing in pigs are observed.

Diagnosis

It is based on history, clinical signs and postmortem lesions described above, and serum or CSF sodium levels. Serum or CSF sodium levels > 150 mmol/L (or mEq/L) is indicative of salt poisoning. Similarly, cerebrum sodium content > 1800 ppm from dead animals is also indicative. Ingesta or urinary sodium content are also useful in correlating the diagnosis for salt toxicity.

Treatment

Prognosis of salt poisoning is often grave. Removing source and providing small quantities of fresh salt-free drinking water at regular short intervals, is key for successful therapy in responding cases. Utmost care should be taken while providing water because sudden supply of large volume of water will aggravate cerebral oedema. Supportive therapy includes use of diuretics like furosemide and non-sodium isotonic or slight hypertonic fluids (5 per cent dextrose) to correct the cerebral oedema. Gastrointestinal and CNS sedatives can be used as per conditions. Fresh water for treatment purpose should be restricted to 0.5 per cent of body weight per hour of interval. Attempts should be made to lower serum sodium level at the rate of 0.5 – 1.0 mEq/L per hour.

Following formula, based on serum sodium monitoring, can be used to know the water requirement to be supplied to affected animal:

Free water deficit (FWD) in Litres = [0.6 x Body weight (in kg) x {(measured serum Na/normal serum Na) -1}]

About 50 per cent of calculated FWD is to be supplied within first 24 h and remaining in following 24-48 h.

4. Fluoride

Fluorine (F) is a halogen element which is unstable and rarely occurs in nature. Its ionic form (F⁻ ion) is known as fluoride which occurs in nature mainly in rocks and soil. Rock-phosphates and ores like fluorspar, cryolite, topaz and mica are rich in sodium or calcium or silicate salts of fluoride. Fluoride is mainly found in calcified tissues in the body and approximately 99 per cent of the fluoride is found in bones and teeth. Fluoride is believed to be an essential mineral in micro-quantities as it enhances strength of tooth enamel by formation of fluorapatite and prevents dental caries. In animals, acute poisoning of fluoride is rare. Fluoride intoxication is mostly observed in chronic form following prolonged ingestion of small quantities of fluoride or its salts, and the resulting toxicosis is known as fluorosis. Thus, the term fluorosis is more common in use and simply refers to chronic fluoride toxicity. Rock phosphate more than 100 ppm or sodium fluoride more than 40 ppm in diet can cause fluoride toxicity in cattle.

The order of species susceptibility for fluorosis is Cattle and Buffalo > Sheep > Horse. Pig and poultry are rarely affected by fluorosis as they have shorter economic life. Young ones in developing skeletal stage are more affected by fluorosis as compared to adults. Dairy cattle are more affected than the beef cattle.

Sources of Poisoning

i. The main source of fluoride toxicity in both animals and humans is the intake of groundwater contaminated by geological sources, or deep bore well waters naturally high in fluoride content. Fluoride level in water as low as 1.5 ppm is able to produce fluorosis in several species.

ii. Sodium fluoride (NaF): It is used to fluoridate water or in fluoridated tooth-pastes. It is also a weak anti-coagulant. In veterinary medicine, it is used as acaricide, pediculicide and ascaricide. It is used as vermifuge in swine and can cause acute fluoride toxicity, if given at levels excess than 4-5 per cent in swine-feed. Sodium fluoride is more soluble and more toxic salt form of fluoride.

iii. Industrial affluent, waste or smoke especially from fertilizer industries and metal purifying units may contain high level of fluorides. Consumption of fodder and water contaminated by the fumes and dusts emitting from superphosphate fertiliser plants may cause fluorosis in livestock. Contaminated fodders containing more than 50 ppm of fluoride predispose to fluorosis in ruminants. Sodium fluorosilicate is a toxic by-product of super-phosphate fertilizers.

iv. Volcanic activities responsible for pasture contamination have beenreported to cause fluoride intoxication in both domestic and wild grazing animals.

Toxicokinetics

Fluoride is rapidly and efficiently absorbed from gastrointestinal tract of animals, both from intestine and stomach. More than 80 per cent of soluble fluoride compounds are absorbed *e.g.* sodium fluoride, hydrogen fluoride, and fluorosilic acid. After absorption, fluoride is rapidly distributed between the plasma and blood cells, with plasma levels being twice as high as blood cell levels. Distribution of fluoride into soft tissues (*e.g.* pineal gland) and calcified tissue readily occurs and is dependent on age. As like for lead, bone acts as sink for fluoride also, as more than 95 per cent of body fluoride got deposited into bone. Fluoride fairly crosses placental barrier but its transfer from plasma to milk is poor. Major route of fluoride excretion from the body is *via* the kidneys; but to a lesser extent, it is also excreted in the faeces, sweat, and saliva.

Toxicodynamics

Acute Fluoride Toxicity

Acute oral LD_{50} of sodium fluoride reported in rat and mouse is reported to be 31 - 101 and 44.3 mg F^-/kg body weight, respectively. Fluoride salts act as strong irritant on GIT causing gastroenteritis. In strong acidic medium of stomach, fluoride forms hydrofluoric acid which produces corrosive effects on GIT. Acute toxicity of fluoride involves binding of fluoride ion to important cations of body like calcium and magnesium resulting in impaired ionic balance like hypocalcaemia, hypomagnesaemia, and hyperkalemia. Hypocalcaemia and hypomagnesaemia causes CNS symptoms and seizures whereas hyperkalemia affects the heart. Formation of calcium fluoride acts as anticoagulant and cause coagulation defects. Fluoride ions also exert direct toxic effects on cellular enzymatic systems.

Fluorosis (Chronic fluoride toxicity)

Mainly, two types of fluorosis lesions are observed in animal *viz. dental fluorosis* and *skeletal fluorosis* (*osteofluorosis*). Fluorosis characterized by mottling and abrasion of teeth, and intermittent lameness. Dental fluorosis is observed if fluorosis strikes at early age in animals for example upto 3 to 4 years in cattle. If exposure occurs at later stages of life, only skeletal form of fluorosis is observed.

Other effects include intermittent diarrhea, weight loss, reduction in milk and wool production, polydipsia, polyuria and aplastic anemia are other significant clinical signs. There is also effect on reproduction in cattle and increased postcalving anestrous is observed in cows having chronic ingestion of diet having 8-12 ppm fluoride.

(A) Dental Fluorosis

It is mainly seen in young animals because fluoride affects erupting teeth in developing stage and damages ameloblast and odontoblast. Young cattle between ages of 6 months to 3 years are affected. There is delayed and irregular defective mineralization leading to malformation of enamel and dentine. Hypoplasia of enamel is observed in severe fluorosis cases. Erosions and pitting of enamel results into fissures or abrasion. Oxidation of organic matrices on surface and deposition of pigments on enamel fissure resulted into brown-black discolouration with alternating white opaque horizontal areas known as mottling of teeth. Dental caries are observed in advanced cases of dental fluorosis.

(B) Skeletal Fluorosis

Osteofluorosis results into disrupted osteogenesis as well as replacement of hydroxyl radicals by fluoride ions in the hydroxyapatite of the bone matrix. Disrupted osteogenesis leads to inadequate matrix formation, poor mineralization and thus, accelerated bone resorption and osteoporosis. In the process of repair, there is abnormal remodeling with collagenous fibers causing abnormal bone growth in form of sclerosis and exostoses. Such growth and fluoride deposition is more on periosteal surface of long bones known as lateral exostoses. Periosteal overgrowth around joints with ossification of ligaments, tendon sheaths and tendons occurs.

Clinical Signs

Dental Fluorosis

Abrasion and mottling of enamel and teeth, discoloration, dental caries, pain while chewing and mastication and sensitiveness due to exposure of pulp cavity, incisor teeth are more affected, decrease in growth and production of animal due to improper mastication and decrease in feed intake. Dental fluorosis was common in buffalo compared to cattle.

Skeletal Fluorosis

Non-specific shifting lameness is observed which means pain, stiffness and lameness is on-going and intermittent in nature over extended period of time. Generally, bilateral and symmetric lesions are seen. Bones primarily affected by fluorosis are mandibles, metatarsal, metacarpal and ribs. Long bones are more prone to fracture. Abnormal hoof wear along with elongated toes particularly in hind-limbs is observed.

Post-mortem Findings

Gastroenteritis, affections of teeth and bone, chalky white appearance of long bones with lateral exostoses, degenerative changes in the bone-marrow (aplastic anemia), central nervous system, cardiac muscles, adrenal glands, liver and kidney. Loop of Henle and collecting tubules of the kidney are affected.

Diagnosis

Other than history, clinical signs and postmortem lesions described above, X-ray and biopsy of rib along with analysis of fluoride in bone and urine are helpful in diagnosis of fluorosis. Increased density of bones is observed. Analysis of fluoride content in feed and water is also useful. In cattle, fluoride (F^-) content > 3000 ppm in bone or 15 ppm in urine is indicative of fluorosis. Higher fluoride content (upto 6000 ppm) in bone is observed for sheep but lower values (500-1000 ppm) are observed for horses affected with fluorosis. Normally cattle bone contains 200–1800 ppm fluoride whereas cattle urine contains less than 6 ppm fluoride. Differential diagnosis for fluorosis should be considered with parathyroid disease, degenerative arthritis, and osteoporosis resulting from deficiency of calcium, phosphorus or vitamin D.

Treatment

Removal of source is important. Mineral supplements and bone meal based feed should be used very cautiously. Water source from deep bore well or artesian bore should be monitored for its fluoride content. Since there is no specific antidote for fluoride toxicity, treatment is mainly symptomatic and supportive. Salts of aluminium and calcium, like aluminium sulfate (30g/d), aluminium chloride or calcium carbonate can bind excess or residual fluoride present in GIT and hence, reduces fluoride absorption.

Chapter 4

Residue Toxicology

☆ *R.D. Singh and V.N. Sarvaiya*

Residue toxicology can be defined as a branch of science which deals with the study of chemical residues in food. It mainly includes the study of sources and quantification of residues, their health impact, setting their tolerance limit and ameliorative or preventive measures to reduce residues in food. Chemical residues in animal origin food are one of the most critical issues in food safety in the perspective of both public health as well as trade concerns. These residues include the residues from pesticides used in agriculture for fodder production and vector control; feed – additives and other growth promoting agents, veterinary drugs *viz.* antimicrobials, anthelmintics, coccidiostats, ectoparasiticides and hormonal agents *etc.,* and sometimes industrial contaminants.

Veterinary drug residue is defined as drugs and their metabolites which are found in the edible tissues including milk of animals after their medication with specific drugs. After medication of an animal, all the drug molecules should be excreted from the animal body through excretion but many drugs and their metabolites are likely to persist in the various tissues of the animal body in low concentrations. This small residual pool of drug and metabolites found in animal products like meat or milk comprise drug residue. The total residue of a drug in animal-derived food consists of the parent drug together with all the metabolites and drug based products that remain in the food after administration of the drug to food-producing animals. The amount of total residue is generally determined by means of a study using the radiolabelled drug and is expressed as the parent drug equivalent in mg/kg of the food. Thus, Total drug residue includes parent compound, metabolites, excipients in the formulation and associated impurities. Residues may be extractable or bound (non-extractable) residues based on their extractability from tissues or biological fluids by exhaustive extraction, denaturation or solubilization techniques.

1. Hazards of Residues

Unlike microbial pathogens of food contamination which constitutes the immediate risk to human health, chemical residues in food mostly cause long-term but serious nature of incidences. Toxicity of pesticide residue includes cancer (carcinogenic agents), chronic renal disorders, reproductive disorders, endocrine disorders (endocrine disruptors), neurological, behavioural and learning disorders and immunosuppression. Adverse effects of veterinary drug residues include:

1. Drug-specific toxicities (depend on intrinsic nature of drug), for example, sulpha drug produce renal toxicity and chloramphenicol produce bone marrow suppression.

2. Drug allergy: Beta-lactam class of antibiotics like penicillin can produce a cutaneous eruption, anaphylaxis and gastrointestinal symptoms in hypersensitive population.

3. Cancer: Some drugs have been found to be carcinogenic in laboratory animals and hence are banned from use in many countries *e.g.* nitrofurans and nitroimidazoles.

4. Adverse effect on beneficial gastrointestinal tract (GIT) microflora of consumer *e.g.* Residues of broad-spectrum antimicrobials like tetracycline.

In addition to these direct thrashings due to pesticide and drug residues, following indirect harms also occur:

1. Development of antimicrobial resistance owing to the selection of resistant (mutant) bacteria and then the transfer of the resistance.

2. Economic loss due to the restrictions on export trade, poor quality or failure of food processing/dairy plant processing, change in organoleptic qualities of food *etc.*

2. Concepts of Withdrawal Time and MRL

Withdrawal Time (or Withdrawl Period)

A withdrawal time is established to safeguard human from exposure to a drug residue in the food. The withdrawal time is the time required for the residue of toxicological concern to reach safe concentration as guided by tolerance limits or maximum residue limit (MRL). In other words, it is the time required after administration of a drug to a food-producing animal, needed to assure that drug residue in the marketable animal product (milk/meat) is below a legally prescribed MRL or in safe concentrations. It is calculated from the time an animal is removed from medication until the permitted time of slaughter for meat producing animals.

It reflects the time required for metabolism and excretion of parent drugs and metabolites (generally marker residues) in such an extent that their concentration in edible tissue becomes under the safe and accepted limit. Marker Residue is residue whose concentration decreases in a known relationship to the level of total residues in milk, meat, eggs, or other animal tissues. A specific and sensitive quantitative analytical method for measuring its concentration is available. Withdrawal time or period of a drug depends on species type of animal product (egg/meat/milk), route of administration (SC/Oral/IM/IV) and type of drug and its formulation (long or short acting formulations).

Good practice in the use of veterinary drugs (GPVD) is the official recommended or authorized usage including withdrawal periods, approved by national authorities, of veterinary drugs under practical conditions.

In the year 2012, an amendment in Sub-rule 3 of rule 97 of Drug and Cosmetic Rules 1945 (under the Drug and Cosmetic Act, 1940) in India, was made which read 'Medicine for food-producing animals shall be labelled with withdrawal period of the drug for the species on which it is intended to be used'. If specific withdrawal period is not mentioned, it should be considered minimum 7 days for milk and 28 days for meat.

Maximum Residue Limit (MRL)

Maximum Residue Limit (MRL) is the maximum concentration of a drug or chemical residue in feed or animal product, resulting from the registered use of a pesticide or drug that is legally permitted by concerned authorities of the respective country. The term 'tolerance limit' is similar phrase mostly used for pesticides and represents upper legal pesticide residue concentration in food based on good agricultural practice.

In India, MRLs for agrochemicals in food products are now regulated by ministry of health and family welfare under Food Safety and Standards (Contaminants, Toxins and Residues) Regulation, 2011. Earlier, MRLs or tolerance limits were specified in Prevention of Food Adulteration (PFA) act, 1955. Food Safety and Standards Authority of India (FSSAI) Act (2006), Sec. 16(2) (6) specify the limit (MRL or Tolerance Limit) for use of food additives, pesticide residues, the residue of Veterinary drugs *etc.* A new pesticide can got registered under central insecticides board and registration committee (CIB and RC) (Insecticide Act, 1968) only if its tolerance limits are specified for its residues under FSSAI, 2006. In absence of an established MRL in India under FSSAI or PFA, MRLs specified in Codex Alimentarius (FAO/WHO) are followed.

For antibacterial drug, other than toxicological MRL which is to be determined by acute, subacute, and medium-term toxicities, genotoxicity, reproductive and embryotoxicity; bacteriological MRL also exists which is determined by NOEL (no observable effect level) on GIT flora multiplication. Generally bacteriological MRL is lower than toxicological MRL.

For setting up of MRL values, acceptable daily intake (ADI) is calculated with NOEL and safety factors. ADI is an estimate of the amount of a chemical agent whose residue is in the question, expressed on a body weight basis that can be ingested daily over a lifetime without appreciable health risk. For ADI standard, weight of man is considered 60 kg. Another important consideration taken into account is average consumption or ingestion per individual of different types of food (milk, meat, vegetables, fruits, cereals *etc.*) in particular country. The NOEL is the highest dose or exposure level of a poison that produces no noticeable toxic effect on animals. Residue tolerance levels that are permitted in food or in drinking water are usually set from 100 to 1,000 times less than the NOEL to provide a wide margin of safety for humans.

MRLs of some Important Pesticides in Milk and Milk Products (Prevention of Food Adulteration Act, now FSS Act, 2006)

Sl.No.	Name of the Pesticide	Tolerance Limit (ppm)
1	Aldrin, Dieldrin, Heptachlor	0.15
2	Chlordane, Carbofuran	0.05
3	DDT	1.25
4	Fenitrothion	0.05
5	Deltamethrin	0.05 (in milk)
6	Chlorpyriphos, Carbendazine, Benomyl	0.10
7	Cypermethrin, 2,4-D	0.20
8	Ethion	0.50
9	Monocrotophos	0.02
10	Trichlorfon	0.1 (in milk)
11	Lindane (gamma- HCH)	0.05 (in milk)
		0.01 (milk product)

Source: Adopted from Reddy and Reddy, 2015.

MRLs (Maximum Residue Levels) of some Important Veterinary Drugs in Bovine Milk (European Commission, 1999)

Sl.No.	Pharmacological Active Substances	Marker Residues	MRLs in milk (µg/kg)
1	All sulfonamide drugs*	Same as parent drug	100
2	Trimethoprim	Trimethoprim	50
3	Amoxicillin, Ampicillin, Benzyl penicillin	Same as parent drug	4
4	Cloxacillin, Dicloxacillin	Same as parent drug	30
5	Cefazoline	Cefazoline	50
6	Cefquinome	Cefquinome	20
7	Enrofloxacin#	Sum of enrofloxacin and its metabolite ciprofloxacin	100
8	Tylosin	Tylosin A	50
9	Chlortetracycline	Sum of parent drug and its 4-epimer	100
10	Oxytetracycline		
11	Thiamphenicol	Thiamphenicol	50
12	Spiramycin	Sum of spiramycin and neospiramycin	200

Sl.No.	Pharmacological Active Substances	Marker Residues	MRLs in milk (µg/kg)
13	Albendazole	Sum of albendazole -sulphoxide, sulphone, and 2-aminosulphone	100
14	Fenbendazole	Sum of extractable residues which may be oxidized to oxfendazole sulphone	10
15	Eprinomectin	Eprinomectin B1a	30
16	Tolfenamic acid	Tolfenamic acid	50
17	Dexamethasone	Dexamethasone	0.3

* The combined total residue of all substances within the sulfonamide group should not exceed 100 µg/kg.

Combined residue of enrofloxacin and ciprofloxacin should not exceed 100 µg/kg.

Withdrawal Period (Milk for human consumption) as Mentioned on the Product Labels of some Veterinary Drugs Available in Indian Market

Sl.No.	Brand Name	Pharmaceutical Active Substances (Drugs)	Manufacturer	Route	Withdrawal Period (Milk)
1	Isoflud	Isoflupredone acetate	Zydus AHL	Inj.	Nil
2	Avil vet	Pheniramine maleate	Merial	IM/IV	7 days
3	Tribivet	Vit.B_1, B_6, B_{12}	Intas Pharma	Inj.	Nil
4	M-ceft	Ceftizoxime	Alembic	Inj.	5 days
5	Inflavet	Meloxicam, Lignocaine HCL, Paracetamol	Virbac	Inj.	5 days
6	Neoprofen	Ketoprofen	Zoetis	IM/IV	7 days
7	Artizone-S	Phenylbutazone sodium slalicyclate	Zoetis	IM	7 days
8	Catosal	Butaphosphan, Cynoco-balamine	Bayer	Inj.	Nil
9	Wofur	Ceftiofur sodium	Vetoquinol	C/H- IM Poultry- SC	Nil
10	Vetmate	Cloprostenol	Provimi	IM	Nil
11	Bactrisol	Sulphadiazine, trimethoprim	Zoetis	Deep IM	17 days
12	Butalex	Buparvaquione	Zydus AHL	IM	48 hrs (2d)
13	Berenil vet RTU	Diminazene aceturate	Intervet	Deep IM	3 days
14	Panacur (bolus)	Fenbendazole	MSD Animal health	Oral	Nil
15	Uddercef	Cefuroxime	Zydus AHL	I/mammary	48 hrs (2d)
16	Mastiwok	Cefoperazone	Vetoquinol	I/mammary	84 hrs
17	Vetalgin vet	Analgin	MSD Animal health	IM/IV	2 days
18	Enrocin	Enrofloxacin	Zoetis	IM	4 days
19	Lixen I.U	Cephalexin	Virbac	I/U	7 days

Sl.No.	Brand Name	Pharmaceutical Active Substances (Drugs)	Manufacturer	Route	Withdrawal Period (Milk)
20	Antrycide Prosalt	Quinapyramine Sulphate and chloride	Virbac	SC	4 days
21	Amoxirum Forte	Amoxicillin sodium Salbactam	Virbac	Inj.	7 days
22	Duraprogen	Hydroxyprogesterone	Vetcare	IM	7 days
23	Feritas	Iron sorbitol, folic acid and Vit. B_{12}	Intas Pharma	IM	Nil
24	Surral	Isometamidium chloride	Alembic	Deep IM	Nil

Zero Withdrawal Drugs

Zero withdrawal drugs are those whose use does not demand to withhold milk/meat after their administration as these drugs do not enter into milk/do not accumulate or persist in the body. Thus, their withdrawal time is zero-day, for example, eprinomectin in milk, ceftiofur in meat *etc.*

Zero Tolerance Drugs

Zero tolerance drugs are those which should not be present in animal products even at nano concentrations as these are very hazardous substances *i.e.* MRL is nearly zero. Rationally, there is no product coming from a treated animal should be consumed unless the entire drug administered has been eliminated. This concept of zero tolerance is equivalent to the idea of the total absence of residual amounts. Zero tolerance drugs are banned in many countries for use in food-producing animals and poultry, for example, there is no approved tolerance for chloramphenicol in food products and any residue detected is considered violative.

3. Minimizing Drugs and Toxic Residues in Animal Products

Following strategies should be adopted for effective management of drug residue catastrophe:

    (a) The very first step towards limiting drug residues in animal products is to make aware the livestock stakeholders including owners and veterinary personnel through effective extension education. Livestock farmers and animal health caretakers should be made aware of compliance with withdrawal period.

    (b) Minimum use of therapeutic drugs should be practised with more focus on better management and preventive measures of animal health.

    (c) Clean milk production with maximum organic farming approach should be encouraged. Ethno-veterinary practices may be promoted.

    (d) Use antimicrobial agents only if necessary and that too with utmost care that proper dosage regimen must be followed.

(e) Recording of treatments and marking of treated animals should be done as pulling of milk from treated animal to that of healthy animals could be avoided.

(f) Rapid screening procedures for the analysis of antibiotic residues and instant grading and development of simple and economic field test to identify drug residue in edible animal products should be developed.

(g) Nationwide monitoring and surveillance of drug residue in edible tissues and milk is needed and already implicated in many countries including India.

Chapter 5

Zootoxins

Vikas Karande and Ashali Karande

Many animals have developed some means of defense system for protection and to get food. These defense systems involve secretion of chemicals which may be hazardous to the other livings of nature. Toxic animals possess a specialized venom system and are able to produce their own venom, which is mixture of proteins and peptide toxins. Every animal kingdom produce poisons or venom to get food, protection or as a defensive act, *i.e. zootoxin.*

The venom (mixture of toxins) typically stored in a discrete gland and a specialized delivery system. A wide range of venom delivery systems have evolved to facilitate the delivery of venoms, including fangs or modified teeth, harpoons, nematocysts, pincers, proboscises, spines, sprays, spurs and stings. The process of delivery of venom is known as envenomation. The common and well known venomous animals include

☆ Cnidarians- *e.g.* Jellyfishes

☆ Mollusks- *e.g.* Snails

☆ Annelids- *e.g.* Leeches

☆ Arthropods- *e.g.* Spiders, scorpions, bees, wasps, ants and ticks

☆ Echinoderms- *e.g.* Starfishes

☆ Vertebrates- *e.g.* Fishes, snakes and lizards

Poisons are generally secondary products of metabolism that gets deposited in the most animal or in predators following ingestion of pray. Hence to deliver such compounds (to other generally requires) salivary or oral contact and sometimes dermal contact is required.

Venoms and poisons are mixtures of different compounds and most of the time they act synergistically to produce toxic effect in target animals, *e.g.*- peptides, amines, serotonins, quinines, polypeptides and several proteins and enzymes. Though envenomation is rare; it is always a emergency conditions and veterinarian have to treat the animal and not the poison or poisonous animals. Some of the common zootoxins producing agents are snakes, spiders amphibians, and some fishes as well as insects *etc.*

1. Snake Venom

Out of the total 3000 species of snakes 375-400 are poisonous. One lac annual death in animals reported worldwide. Annually around 1.5 to 2 million peoples get bitten by snakes (venomous or non-venomous), whereas deaths reported are around 50,000 or more. Highly venomous snakes observed in Australia but more deaths of humans or animals found in Asian countries like Srilanka, India and Pakistan. There are two types of snake families:

1. Elapine (Elapidae family)- Cobras, Kraits, Coral snakes and Australian adder. The venom of these is neurotoxic and kills the victim by paralysis of respiratory centers.

2. Viperine: Vipers, Russel's viper and English adder. Their venom is haemotoxic and causes intense local damage.

All the venoms have both neurotoxins and haemotoxins, only the quantity varies. The toxic principles in venom are: hyaluronidase, cholinesterase, proteolytic phosphatases and neurotoxins.

Amongst the animals, dogs are most susceptible followed by horses. Cats are resistant. Large animals are mainly bitten on limbs and face and they rarely die, as large quantity of poison or venom is required for death of animals.

The order of susceptibility of different domestic animals is as horses > sheep > cattle> goat > dog > pig > Cat.

Most Venomous Snakes

Type of Snake	Features
Cobra ☆ King cobra (*Ophiophagus hannah*) ☆ Asiatic cobra (*Naja naja*) ☆ Egyptian cobra (Naja haje)	☆ Found near the human and animal shelters, and in agriculture farms. ☆ Sometime found in cultivated land in search of rodents. ☆ Deep fang marks may be observed at site. ☆ Highly neurotoxic and death occur due to respiratory failure. Venom is sufficient to kill adult elephant. ☆ Only snake who built a shelter for laying eggs.
Indian Krait	☆ Fifteen times more deadly then common cobra. ☆ Powerful venom is powerful neurotoxic. Death occurs due to respiratory failure. ☆ Easily comes under foot.

Type of Snake	Features
Vipers	☆ Highly aggressive and bite immediately.
☆ Pit Viper (*Trimeresurus gramineus*)	☆ Produce rasping sound by rubbing its body.
☆ Habu pit viper	☆ Usually found many bite marks at bite site due to chewing.
☆ Saw scaled viper	
☆ Russell's Viper (*Vipera russellii*)	☆ Venom is highly hemotoxic.
	☆ Venom causes intense pain, swelling, bleeding, lowers blood pressure and heart rate.
	☆ Most of the times it bites at head and shoulder regions. Causes intense pain and death.

Mechanism of Action

☆ α toxin in cobra causes irreversible neuromuscular blocking by acting on nicotinic receptors and death is due to failure of cellular respiration getting affected.

☆ Causes paralysis of somatic motor nerves.

☆ Hemotoxin causes hemolysis.

☆ All toxins cause hepatic and renal damage.

Symptoms

Initially there is restlessness and intense local pain, swelling, however in cobra bite there is no swelling. The animal becomes excited, pupils get dilated, gasping, salivation and later depression, in coordination and collapse. Skin is cold. There is no response to external stimuli, paralysis of tongue, cyanosis, convulsions and death. In hemotoxins there is hemolysis and hemoglobinuria is observed. In case of small animals there may be decreased temperature and vomition is seen.

Diagnosis

Diagnosis can be done on the basis of history, local swelling at the site of bite and presence of fang marks. History of snakes in the vicinity of animals shelter is a key point.

Treatment

The snake bite cases must attended immediately and fast treatment should be initiated so the survival chances will increase. Movement of animal should be restricted to reduce the absorption of venom hence animal should be rested. If medical aid not possible, immediately first aid should be initiated.

    i. First aid- Initially cleaning and washing of the wound with alkaline soap should be initiated. Tourniquet should be applied 2- 4 inches above the wound site so as to reduce absorption. Tourniquet should be released after some time and arterial flow should not be obstructed. Take shallow cuts with aseptic blade and apply suction to remove the venom.

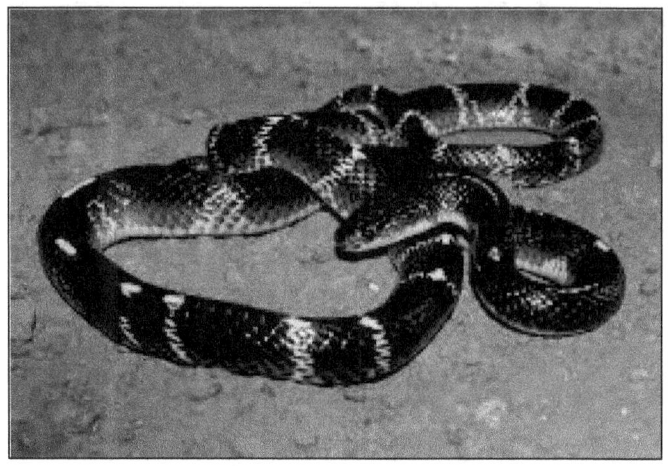

Common Krait – (*Bungarus Caeruleus*).

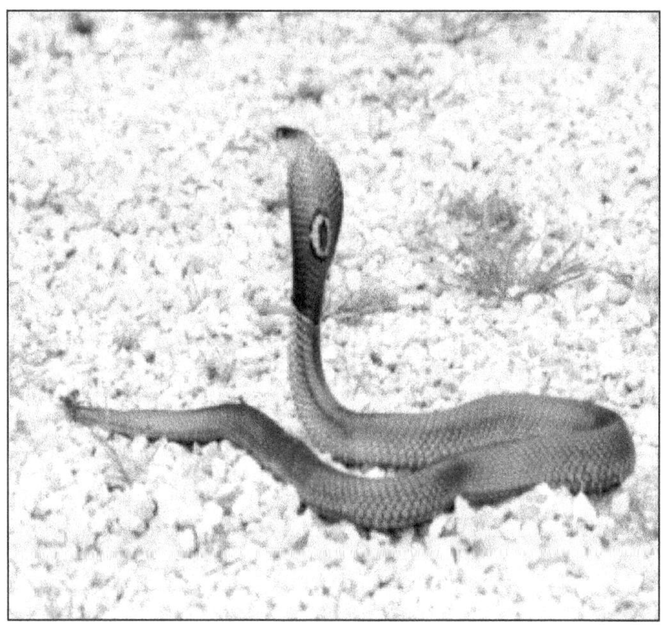

Indian Cobra.

ii. Specific treatment- Monovalent Snake antivenin is useful if the snake is known otherwise use polyvalent antisnake venom serum. Large quantity is given by I/V or S/C or I/P route in 5 per cent dextrose solution.

☆ For large animals: 2 Units per 150 kg body weight

☆ For small animals: 10 Units per 20-40 kg body weight

In human beings anaphylactic actions due to serum are noted, but rare in animals.

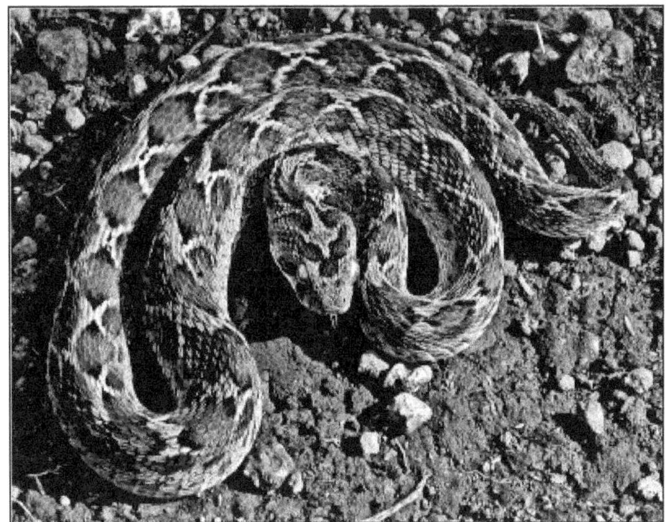

Saw Scaled Viper.

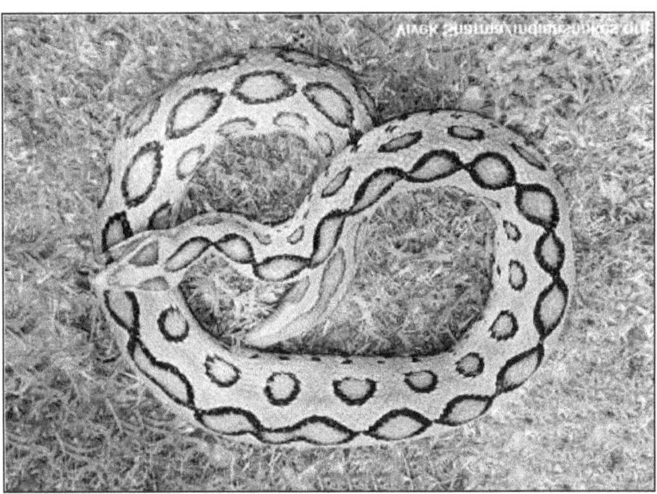

Russel's Viper.

iii. Supportive treatment- Broad spectrum antibiotics, blood transfusion or saline. Give serum along with epinephrine to reduce anaphylaxis. Give corticosteroids. Calcium gluconate prevents haemolysis.

iv. Do not give hot and cold applications, no antihistamines and do not wash with $KMnO_4$.

2. Scorpion Venom

These are arachnids and body consisting of head and thorax with four pairs of legs. A barbed appendage called telson bearing two venomous glands. Scorpions hide in dark spaces like inside shoes, under rocks, or inside vegetation. Scorpions found all over the globe. Scorpions are opportunistic predators of small arthropods and insects. The Red and Black Indian scorpions are listed as most dangerous scorpions, around 10-20 peoples die by scorpion bite in a year in India. Scorpion sting is an acute life-threatening, time-limiting medical emergency in rural areas. However in case of animals it is mostly unnoticed. Numerous envenomations are unreported and true incidence is not known. Reported fatality rates are of 3-22 per cent among children hospitalized for scorpion stings in India, Saudi Arabia and South Africa. However, reports on fatality rates in animals are rare.

In India, among 86 scorpion species *Mesobuthus tamulus* and *Palamneus swammer-dami* are of medical importance. Stings may cause cardiovascular effects. Scorpions live in warm dry regions throughout India. They inhabit commonly the crevices of dwellings, underground burrows, under logs or debris, paddy husk, sugarcane fields, coconut and banana plantations. Their distribution is more in regions with abundant red soil. Stings are mostly in summer as compared to winter season primarily due to accidental contact with scorpion.

Mechanism of Action

Venom is generally consisting low molecular weight polypeptides. They block the voltage sensitive Sodium and Potassium channels.

Symptoms

Intense generalized pain and edema which may lasts for several hours, enlarged lymph nodes, allergic reactions, swelling around the eyes, swollen face are prominently seen. It is neurotoxic venom and has hyaluronidase, 5-HT, hexosamine

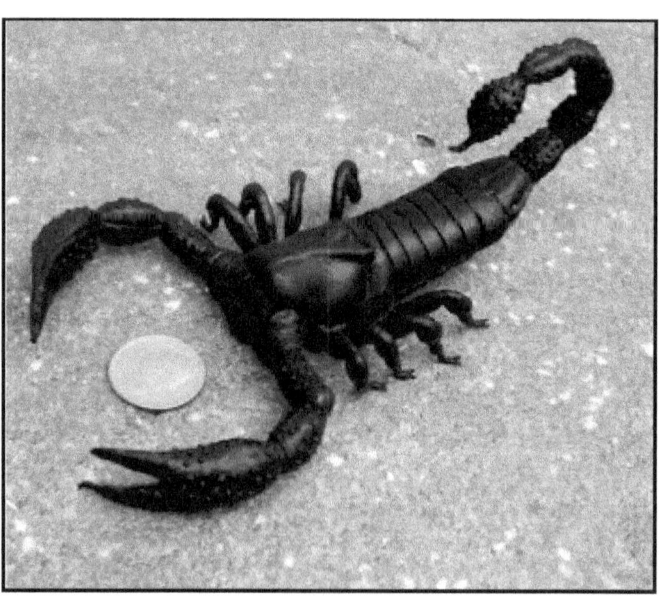

Scorpion.

and kinin. After bite there is local swelling, intense pain, and convulsions due to persistent depolarization. Tachycardia seen within 4 hours and persist upto 24-72 hours. Tachycardia, hypertension, myocardial dysfunction, pulmonary edema and shock is spectrum of one process *viz.*, autonomic storm. Death occurs rarely.

Treatment

Treatment is mostly symptomatic. Prazosin is useful to neutralize the effects of an over stimulated autonomic nervous system. Scorpion antivenins, if available will be helpful. Scorpion venoms reach their target too rapidly to be neutralized and antivenin within 30 minutes of sting may reverse their effect.

3. Spider

About 35,000 species of spiders described worldwide, out of these 27 species are considered to be dangerous have caused fatalities. Spiders are distributed everywhere and having 8 segmented legs, and two segmented body. Their habitation is mostly in dark area, dense growing plants, under appliances and cabinets. Spider bite may cause swelling and intense pain, anaphylaxis and other allergic reactions. They produces mostly two type of toxicity *i.e.*, neurotoxic (affects the central nervous system) and cytotoxic effect (affects the tissue around the bite site). There are many types of spider found all over the world.

a. Black Widow Spider (*Latrodectus mactans*)- found in south of united states

b. Western Black Widow Spider (*L. herperus*)- common in western U.S.

c. Northern widow spider (*L. varioles*)

d. Red widow spider (*L. bishepi*)

e. Brown widow spider (*L. geomatrius*)

Mechanism of Action

Spider releases mixture of neuroactive proteins and proteolytic enzymes. Latrotoxine is polypeptide in nature which generally causes heavy release of acetylcholine and nor-epinephrine initially and later their depletion at post

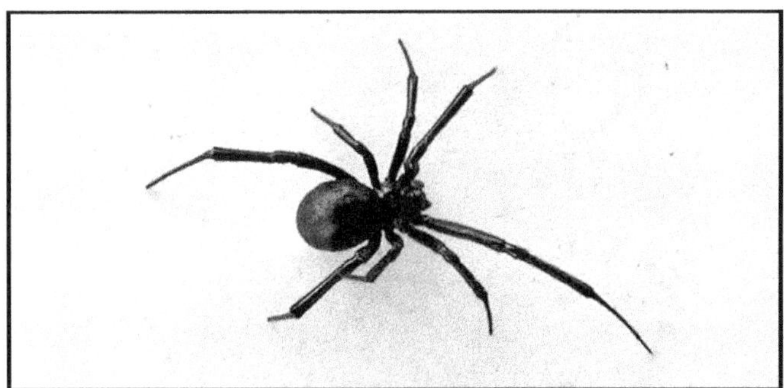

Black Widow Spider.

ganglionic sympathetic synapses. It is highly toxic and LD_{50} value is 0.9 mg/Kg in mice. After the bite the Venom is taken up by bloodstream through lymphatics.

After initial pain, swelling at site starts up to 30 minutes. Later pain spreads to all over body within 2 to 3 hrs. Tachycardia is a common syndrome. Generally victim gets relief only after 60 to 72 hrs. But other signs of weakness fatigue may take weeks to subside.

Clinical Signs

Cats and dogs generally are most susceptible because of playing habit with moving objects. May causes paralysis, howling and barking behavior. Swelling, itching, pain, observe for redness spreading away from the bite, watery drainage from the bite, increase in pain, numbness, tingling, and discoloration around the bite. There may severe pain, jelly like edema, emesis, abdominal rigidity, dyspnoea, paralysis and death, within 4 - 6 hours of bite. Other signs may involve restlessness, vomiting, muscle tremors, ataxia, cramps and hyper salivation.

Treatment

Treatment is mostly symptomatic

Prevention

Regular cleaning of animal sheds and restrict entry of pets in dark spaces.

4. Toad Poisons

The toxins secreted from some species of frogs are so strong that simply touching those tiny amphibians can be deadly. The skin of these venomous amphibians has provided with over 400 alkaloids such as the batrachotoxin,

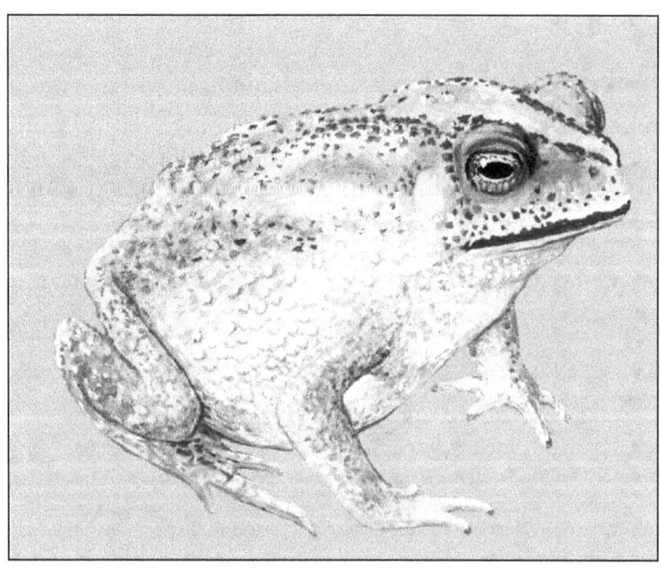

Toad.

histrionic toxins, pumiliotoxin and epibatidine. Poisonous toads are *Bufo vulgaris* (least toxic), common toad and *B. marinus* (most toxic).

Their venom consists of cardiac glycosides (Bufogenin and Bufotoxin), neurotoxin (Bufotoxin), and indol derivatives (Bufotenine and Serotonin). Neurotoxin causes persistent depolarization and paralysis. Secretions also contain histamine, tyramine and catacholamines. Venom is present in skin and stored in parotid gland. Poisoning in dogs is due to contact or ingestion. Symptoms include salivation, in coordination, excitability, tremors, paralysis and death. Treatment is mostly symptomatic.

5. Bees, Wasp and Hornets

No statistics is available for lethal bees or wasp stings in animals. Over 20,000 species found throughout the world. Stinger is the modification of ovipositor apparatus and is found only in female bees and wasps. Venom from specialized cells is transported to the venous sac through small tubules. The stinger of the honey bee is covered with retrograde barks that cause stinger to remain impaled in thick skinned victims. While withdrawing, entire stinger apparatus gets separated from bee which cause death of honey bee. Similar to spiders, venom of honey bee is a complex mixture of proteins, polypeptides and small molecules.

Bee's venom contains histamine and peptides (like apamine and melitin). Wasp venom contains histamine, serotonin, and kinin whereas hornet venom contains histamine, serotonin and acetylcholine. However, hyaluronidase and phospholipase are common in all these venoms. Hyaluronidases present in venom are responsible for allergic reactions whereas; serotonin, histamine, tyramine and acetylcholine are mainly responsible for pain

Sign and symptoms of sting cause intense local pain, local edema, burning, extreme bites excitement, hemoglobinuria, jaundice, and respiratory distress.

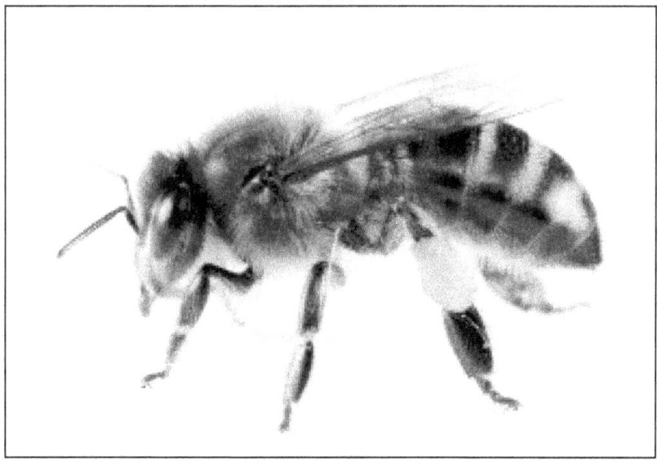

Honey Bee.

Death is due to anaphylactic reactions. Treatment is mainly symptomatic and local application of NH_3 or $NaHCO_3$.

6. Tick Toxins

Common ticks are Dermacentor, Haemaphysalis, Ixodes and Rhipicephalus. Ticks carry their toxins in salivary glands. Toxin causes decrease in release of acetylcholine which may leads to paralysis in lamb, calves and kids. Ticks acts as a vectors for diseases in large member of diseases in animals and human.

All ruminants and pets are susceptible to tick toxins. Toxin interferes with the synthesis and release of neurotransmitter such as acetylcholine at neuromuscular junction. Resulting in paralysis sometimes paralysis of respiratory muscles leads to respiratory failure and death. Symptoms include ascending paralysis and death (due to respiratory failure) is rare. Treatment include removal of ticks and supportive treatment should be provided.

7. Fish Toxins

Several aquatic species carry toxins in their body and the common known example is Puffer fish which is known for its tetrodotoxin. Poisonings from tetrodotoxin have been almost exclusively associated with the consumption of puffer fish from waters of the Indo-Pacific ocean regions, but puffer fishes from other regions are much less commonly eaten. Several reported cases of poisonings, including fatalities, involved puffer fish from the Atlantic Ocean, Gulf of Mexico, and Gulf of California. It is extremely toxic, oral median lethal dose (LD_{50}) in mice is 334 µg per kg body weight. Poisoning occur as a consequence of consumption of fish from the order Tetraodontiformes. Puffer fish contain tetrodotoxin which is sufficient to produce paralysis of the diaphragm and death due to respiratory failure. Toxicity varies on species, seasons, geographic localities. All puffer fish are not equally toxic.

Tetrodotoxin inhibits the firing of action potentials in nerves by binding to the voltage gated sodium channels in nerve cell membranes and block the passage of sodium ions (responsible for the rising phase of an action potential) into the nerve cell. The nervous system fails to carry messages and thus muscles from flexing in response to nervous stimulation.

Diagnosis

Diagnosis should be made on the basis of history of recent consumption of fish and symptoms of toxicity.

Symptoms

Signs of toxicity may be observed after half an hour to four hours of consumption of toxin. Symptoms include hypersalivation, sweating, headache, incoordination, tremor, weakness and lethargy and developing parasthesia of lips tongue and extremities. There may be paralysis, cyanosis, dysphagia and seizures. Gastrointestinal disorders like nausea, vomiting diarrhea and colic may be observed.

Treatment

There is no specific antidote, however, supportive and symptomatic treatment should be intiated immediately. Treatment involves airway management. If toxin is ingested, treatment should consist of emptying the stomach, feeding the victim activated charcoal to bind the toxin, and taking standard life-support measures to keep the victim alive until the effect of the poison disappears.

Saxitoxin

Saxitoxin is a neurotoxin, naturally produced by certain species of marine dinoflagellates and freshwater cyanobacteria. Saxitoxin is a neurotoxin that acts as a selective sodium channel blocker. It is one of the most potent known natural toxins, acting on the voltage-gated sodium channels of neurons, preventing normal cellular function and leading to paralysis. Its oral LD_{50} in mice is 263 µg per kg and for humans it is 5.7 µg per kg. The human illness associated with ingestion of harmful levels of saxitoxin is known as paralytic shellfish poisoning (PSP). Paralytic shellfish poisoning can be fatal in extreme cases, particularly in immunocompromised individuals. Children are more susceptible. PSP affects those who come into contact with the affected shellfish by ingestion.

Symptoms appears within 10-30 minutes of ingestion, and include nausea, vomiting, diarrhea, abdominal pain, tingling or burning lips, gums, tongue, face, neck, arms, legs, and toes. Shortness of breath, dry mouth, a choking feeling and loss of coordination are also possible. Diagnosis on the basis of history, symptoms and also may be made by using radioimmunoassay or ELISA testing.

There are no known antidotes for this type of poisoning so will prefer symptomatic treatment. Shift animal to good ventilated area to get aerolized saxitoxins out of respiratory tract and reduce irritation. Activated charcoal, only if saxitoxins has localized in the intestines may be useful if administered within first two hours of ingestion. If after three hours, the toxin may got passed through the upper digestive tract, then catharsis (vomiting or purging) is recommended.

Chapter 6

Photosensitization and Lathyrism

☆ *Jeevan Ranjan Dash*

Photosensitization

Photosensitization refers to inflammation of the skin and sometimes the conjunctiva and cornea of the eye. It occurs when skin/areas lacking significant protective hair, wool, or pigmentation exposed to sunlight and becomes more susceptible to UV rays because of the presence of photodynamic agents. Photosensitization differs from sunburn in the sense that it does not require prolonged exposure to sunlight to develop. Primary photosensitization occurs due to eating a range of plants that contain photosensitizing substances. Secondary photosensitization occurs due to damage to liver. Photosensitization is more likely to be seen in livestock with unpigmented or white skin. Most susceptible animals are cattle, sheep, goats, and horses.

When photosensitizing substances accumulate in the bloodstream, they may be exposed to sunlight when passing through capillaries close to the surface of the skin, conjunctiva, cornea and other visible mucous membranes. They are activated by the sunlight and cause local tissue damage and inflammation.

Types of Photosensitization

Photosensitization mainly categorized into:

☆ Type-I: Primary photosensitization

☆ Type-II: Secondary/Hepatogenous photosensitization

Type I: Primary Photosensitization

This occurs when the photodynamic agent is ingested, injected, or absorbed through the skin. The photodynamic agent enters the systemic circulation in native form, and on exposure to UV light it damages the skin cell membrane. Some important primary photosensitizing agents are:

- ☆ St John's wort (*Hypericum perforatum*; contains the photosensitizing substance hypericin)
- ☆ Queen Anne's lace (*Ammi majus*; contains furanocoumarins)
- ☆ Buckwheat (*Fagopyrum esculentum*; contains fagopyrin)
- ☆ Parsley (*Petroselinum crispum*; contains furanocoumarins).
- ☆ Coal tar derivatives such as polycyclic aromatic hydrocarbons, tetracyclines, and some sulfonamides have been reported to cause primary photosensitization.
- ☆ Phenothiazine anthelmintics have been reported to cause primary photosensitivity in cattle, sheep, goats, and swine.

Type II: Secondary/Hepatogenous Photosensitization

Secondary photosensitization is the most common form of this disease. It occurs following liver damage from consuming plant toxins. The photosensitising compound is phylloerythrin, produced by the breakdown of chlorophyll in the gastrointestinal tract. Normally, phylloerythrin is absorbed into the blood, then removed by the liver and excreted in the bile. When there is liver damage, this process is disrupted, leading to accumulation of phylloerythrin in the blood and subsequent photosensitization. Secondary photosensitization is most commonly associated with livestock grazing of following plants:

- ☆ Caltrop (*Tribulus terrestris*)
- ☆ *Brachiaria* spp.
- ☆ *Panicum* spp.
- ☆ Ryegrass pastures heavily contaminated with the spores of *Pithomyces chartarum*
- ☆ Rough dog's tail (*Cynosurus echinatus*), leading to acute bovine liver disease
- ☆ Lantana (*Lantana camara*) (only a garden plant in WA).

Signs of Photosensitization

- ☆ Severe irritation, restlessness, rubbing and shaking of head and ears
- ☆ Seeking shade
- ☆ Swelling of affected areas including ears, eyelids, lips and nose. Swelling around the lips and nose may cause difficulty with eating and breathing. Swollen ears droop and may be a distinctive feature
- ☆ Discharge from the eyes, conjunctivitis, corneal opacity
- ☆ Sometimes lameness (photosensitization affecting the coronary band)

☆ Dead and sloughing skin in the affected areas, with underlying tissues becoming inflamed and scabs forming over the inflammation. This is often first noticed at the tips of the ears, but can extend to the whole face, unpigmented areas of the body, and areas of bare skin like the udder, teats, vulva and upper surface of the tail.

☆ Jaundice (yellowing of skin, gums and whites of the eyes) may be noticed in cases of secondary photosensitization.

Diagnosis

Diagnosis of photosensitization is based on clinical signs, evidence or history of exposure to photosensitizing agents or hepatotoxins, and characteristic lesions. Photophobia in combination with erythema and edema of hairless, nonpigmented areas of skin is strongly suggestive of the disease and a definitive diagnosis can be made by measuring porphyrin levels in blood, feces, and urine.

Differential Diagnosis

Diseases have signs that resemble photosensitization are dermatophilosis, scabby mouth, bluetongue disease, foot-and-mouth disease, sheep pox.

Treatment

☆ Remove affected livestock from the toxic plant and provide shade. Housing is preferred for shade cover, rather than trees. Affected livestock will need protection from sunlight for at least seven days.

☆ Corticosteroids, given parenteral injection in the early stages, may be helpful. Secondary skin infections and suppurations should be treated with basic wound management techniques with fly repellant.

☆ With secondary photosensitization, do not feed green or high-protein feeds. Provide only good quality hay with limited amounts of grain. Recovery may take 4–6 weeks.

Lathyrism

Lathyrism is a disease caused by eating seeds of species of Lathyrus (the grass pea), mainly *L. sativus* (the chickpea or khesari), *L. cicera* (flat-podded vetch) and *L. clymenum* (Spanish vetchling). It affects mostly people in Bangladesh, India, Pakistan, Nepal and Algeria but is sometimes also recorded in France, Italy, Spain and Australia. It affects mostly horses and cattle including man. Domestic animals, notably the horse, develop hind limb paralysis after prolonged feeding on lathyrus fodder. Outbreak of the disease usually occurs at times of drought or famine because it flourishes in conditions of both flood and drought, when no other food crop survives.

Beta-oxalyl-amino-L-alanine acid (BOAA), an excitatory neurotoxin which is a glutamate agonist, has been identified in Lathyrus species responsible for the disease. BOAA appears to exert its effects through mitochondrial toxicity causing cell death, especially in motor neurons.

Symptoms

Two forms of lathyrism is seen, Osteolathyrism and neurolathyrism characterized by skeletal deformities and neurodegenerative disorders respectively. Osteolathyrism affects skeletal development: cartilages and bones grow abnormally leaving the body deformed. Walking difficulties, Unbearable cramps, Leg weakness, Spastic paralysis develops which becomes irreversible. A unique symptom of lathyrism is the atrophy of gluteal muscles (buttocks). The toxin may also cause aortic aneurysm where the toxin changes the elasticity of the aorta causing aortic aneurysm that may rupture and causes death.

Management

Eating the Lathyrus fodder with grain having high concentrations of sulphur-based amino acids reduces the risk of lathyrism. Leaching of the fodder with water reduces the toxicity as the toxin is soluble in water.

Treatment

The disease is usually nonprogressive but irreversible. There is no much advance in treatment of this condition. However, centrally acting muscle relaxants like tolperisone can be tried for symptomatic relief.

Chapter 7

Radiation Hazard and Toxicity

☆ *Tariq Ahmad Wani and Naveen Kumar*

Radiation is energy in the form of waves or particles that is emitted from an element. Different sources of radiation include, nuclear weapons, nuclear power plants, radioactive wastes, radioactive materials, industry and diagnostic and therapeutic purposes. Animals are constantly exposed to low levels of naturally occurring radiation called background radiation. Background radiation comes from cosmic radiation and from radioactive elements in the air, water, and ground. Cosmic radiation is concentrated at the poles by the earth's magnetic field and is attenuated by the atmosphere. Thus, exposure is greater for organism living at high latitudes. In addition to naturally occurring radioisotopes, a large number of radioisotopes are produced artificially by nuclear reactors. In the study of toxicity due to radioactivity, it is necessary to know the type of radiation, energies of these radiations and the number of radiation emitted per unit time.

Each radioactive element has more than one isotope. Some isotopes are stable whose configuration does not change with time, and others are called unstable isotopes. Unstable radioisotopes (nuclides) disintegrate (decay) by emitting ionizing radiation alpha (α), beta (β) and gamma (γ). There are about 275 stable isotopes present in nature. Out of those uranium and thorium have only long lived radioactive isotopes. Radioisotope like ^{3}H and ^{14}C are being continuously formed by cosmic rays induced nuclear reactions and are present in nature.

Radiation is detected by measuring the effects produced by its interaction with matter. Radiation detectors can be classified based on the detector material used and/or type of measurement that can be made, *e.g.*, gas filled detectors, scintillation detectors, semiconductor detectors, neutron detectors, *etc.* For measurement and characterization of radiations, it is necessary to understand the interaction of particular radiations with detector material through which they are passing.

Measurement of Radiation

Conventional units of measurement include the roentgen, rad and rem. The roentgen (R) is a unit of exposure, measuring the ionizing ability of x-rays or gamma radiation in air. The radiation absorbed dose (rad) is the amount of that radiation energy absorbed per unit of mass. In International System (SI) units, rad is replaced by gray (Gy) and rem by sievert (Sv).

☆ 1 Gy = 100 rad, and

☆ 1 Sv = 100 rem.

The rad and rem (and hence Gy and Sv) are essentially equal (*i.e.*, the quality factor equals 1) when describing x-rays or gamma or beta radiation.

The amount (quantity) of radioactivity is expressed in terms of the number of nuclear disintegrations (transformations) per second. The becquerel (Bq) is the SI unit of radioactivity; one Bq is 1 disintegration per second (dps). In the US system, one curie is 37 billion Bq.

Classification of Radiations

Radiation is often categorized into ionizing and non-ionizing depending on the energy of the radiated particles. Non-ionizing radiation does not carry enough energy to ionize atoms or molecules. Examples of non ionizing radiation include infrared, thermal radiation, microwaves and radio waves. Ionizing radiation has a higher frequency and shorter wavelength than non-ionizing radiation.

(A) Ionizing Radiation

☆ Alpha (α) radiation

☆ Beta (β) radiation

☆ Gamma (γ) radiation

☆ X- and γ- rays radiation

(B) Non-ionizing Radiation

☆ Ultraviolet (UV-rays) radiation

☆ Infrared radiation

☆ Microwave radiation

☆ Radio or Television waves

☆ Visible light

Ionizing radiation has many uses in treatment and research field but can be a health hazard. Using ionizing radiation requires elaborate radiological protection measures which in generally are not required for non-ionizing radiation.

A common source of ionizing radiation is radioactive materials that emit α, β, γ and other sources of ionizing radiation include x-rays from radiography examinations. Ultraviolet (UV) radiation has features of both ionizing and non-ionizing radiation. While the part of the ultraviolet radiation that penetrates the Earth's atmosphere is non-ionizing, this may cause injury to biological systems by heating effects (*e.g.*, sunburn). Injury of tissue depending on different factors such as radiation dose, rate of exposure, type of radiation, and part of the body exposed. Symptoms may be local (*e.g.*, burns) or systemic (*e.g.*, acute radiation sickness).

(a) Ionizing Radiation

Alpha Particles (α-rays)

These are energetic helium nuclei emitted by some radionuclide with high atomic numbers (*e.g.*, plutonium, radium, uranium). They do not penetrate the outer layers of dead skin cells and cause no damage to the live tissues below (< 0.1 mm). It may dangerous when alpha emitting radioisotopes are ingested or inhaled. A thin paper can stop these α-rays. Alpha particles lose energy rapidly while passing through a medium, because of their relative high specific ionization, and can be stopped even by very thin sheet of paper or thin (less than 0.3 mm) aluminium foil.

Beta Particles (β-rays)

These are more penetrating than alpha particles, but less than gamma. These particles can penetrate more deeply into skin (1 to 2 cm) and cause both epithelial and sub-epithelial damage. Beta particle can penetrate much deeper than that of an alpha particle. This is due to its smaller mass, charge and higher velocity as compared to that of an alpha particle of similar energy. Beta particles with energy above 70 KeV penetrate the dead layer of the skin. Thus β radiation is an external radiation hazard. They can be stopped with aluminium foils. Thickness of foil required for stopping β- rays depends upon their energy.

Gamma Radiation (γ-rays)

This is very short electromagnetic radiation wavelength that can penetrate deeply into tissue (many centimeters). Gamma radiation consists of photons with a wavelength less than 3×10^{-11} meters. While some photons deposit all their energy in the body, other photons of the same energy may only deposit a fraction of their energy and others may pass completely through the body without interacting. The high doses of γ rays also kill body cells and this forms the basis of cancer treatment with cobalt (^{60}Co) and cesium (^{137}Cs) gamma rays sources. Low energy gamma rays are more readily attenuated. Thick lead or concrete sheets are needed to stop them.

Type of Radiation	Energies of Radiation	Range in Air
α-rays	4 to 8 MeV	centimetre
β-rays	Few KeV to 4 MeV	~3 meter
X- and γ-rays	Few KeV to several MeV	not attenuated by air

Ultraviolet Radiation (UV-rays)

Wavelength varies from 10 nm to 125 nm. The sun is a major source of *UV-rays*. They ionize air molecules. UV-rays are strongly absorbed by air and ozone (O_3). Although present in space, reach organisms on living Earth's surface. There is a zone of the atmosphere (ozone layer), starts at about 32 km and extends upward, which absorbs about 98 per cent of non-ionizing radiation. Some ultraviolet spectrum that reaches the ground and causes damage to biological molecules by means of unwanted reactions. An example is formation of pyrimidine dimers in DNA, which begins at wavelengths below 365 nm. This property indicates the dangers of ionizing radiation in biological systems. On the basis of amount of energy they contain and their effects on biological matter, UV-rays can be subdivided into three different wavelength bands such as UV-A, UV-B, and UV-C. UV-C is most energetic and most harmful while UV-A is least energetic and least harmful.

Neutrons

These are electrically neutral particles emitted by a few radionuclides like californium (Cf^{251}) and nuclear fission reactions (in nuclear reactors). Their depth of tissue penetration varies from a few millimeters to several centimeters, depending on their energy. They collide with the nuclei of stable atoms, resulting in emission of energetic protons, alpha and beta particles, and gamma radiation.

(b) Non-Ionizing Radiation

Non-ionizing radiation is too small to produce charged ions when passing through matter. These include radio waves, microwaves and infrared. The lower frequencies of ultraviolet light may cause chemical changes and molecular damage similar to ionization, but is technically not ionizing. The occurrence of ionization depends on the energy of the individual particles or waves, and not on their number. Non-ionizing radiations is an electromagnetic radiation that does not carry enough energy to ionize atoms or molecule. It is thought to be harmless below the level that causes only heating.

Mechanism of Action

Biological effects of radiation result from both direct and indirect action of radiation. Direct action is based on direct interaction between radiation particles and complex body cell molecules (*e.g.*, direct breakup of DNA molecules). Indirect action is more complex and depends heavily on the loss of energy by radiation in the body tissue and the subsequent chemistry.

The most fundamental effect of ionizing radiation on biological molecules is the ionization of water molecules and formation of free radicals (H^+ and OH^-) which react with cellular macromolecule. The interaction of these free radicals with cellular macromolecules such as nucleic acids, proteins, lipids, carbohydrates leads to a sequence of damage like DNA break, point mutation and chromosomal aberrations with subsequent loss of gene products depends on the kind of alteration and can cause cancer or long term genetic alterations.

Factors affecting Radio-Toxicity

  i. *Dose of radiation:* Larger the dose of radition, greater will be the toxicity.

 ii. *Type of radiation:* Ionizing ration are more toxic than non-ionizing radiations.

iii. *Duration of radiation exposure:* Greater the duration of exposure, more will be the toxicity.

 iv. *Health status of animals:* Weak and emaciated animals are sensitive to radio-toxicity.

  v. *Age:* Young and old persons and animals are more radiosensitive than young one.

 vi. *Cell cycle:* Cells are least sensitive when in the 'S' phase, then the G_1 phase, then the G_2 phase and most sensitive in the 'M' phase of the cell cycle. Hence, the order of sensitivity of the cell cycle is M phase > G_2 phase > G_1 phase > S phase.

vii. *Stage of development:* Developing organism (*e.g.*, embryo and fetus) is more radiosensitive.

viii. *Type of tissue:* Tissues with low rates of cell turnover are less sensitive to radiation (*e.g.,* lung, basal layer of skin). Tissues with high rates of cell turnover are highly sensitive to radiation (*e.g.*, stem cell, intestinal epithelium, haemopoietic system, spermatogonia cell, oocytes).

Signs and Symptoms

Clinical manifestations depend on whether radiation exposure involves the whole body (*i.e.*, acute radiation syndrome) or is limited to a small portion of the body (*i.e.*, focal radiation injury). The severity of radiation injury depends on the dose and the length of time over which it is delivered. A single rapid dose is more damaging than the same dose given over weeks or months.

Young animals are more susceptible to radiation injury because they have a higher rate of cellular proliferation. In general, cells that are undifferentiated and those that have high mitotic rates (*e.g.*, stem cells, cancer cells) are particularly vulnerable to radiation. Cellular sensitivities in approximate descending order from most to least sensitive are lymphoid cells > germ cells > proliferating bone marrow cells > intestinal epithelial cells > epidermal stem cells > hepatic cells > epithelium of lung alveoli and biliary passages > kidney epithelial cells > endothelial cells (pleura and peritoneum) > connective tissue cells > bone cells > muscle, brain, and spinal cord cells.

Diagnosis

Diagnosis is by history of exposure, symptoms and signs, and sometimes use of radiation detection equipment to localize and identify radionuclide contamination.

Prognosis is initially estimated by the time between exposure and symptom onset, the severity of those symptoms, and by the lymphocyte count during the initial 24 to 72 h.

Postmortem Findings

☆ Presence of radioactive materials in all soft tissue, organ, bone.

☆ Gastroenteritis haemorrhagic to ulcerative

☆ Ulceration of pharyngeal mucosa

☆ Pulmonary oedema

☆ Fibrinous pericarditis

☆ Degenerative change of bone marrow

Treatment

There is no specific treatment for radiation intoxication. Give only the symptomatic treatment along with supportive therapy and minimize the radiation exposure and contamination.

Prevention and Management

Protection from radiation exposure is accomplished by avoiding contamination with radioactive material, minimizing the duration of exposure, maximizing the distance from the source of radiation, shielding the source and administration of radio protective drugs.

Management focuses on associated traumatic injuries, decontamination, supportive measures, and minimizing exposure. Typical sequence and priorities are under taken for external decontamination like removing clothing and external debris, decontaminating wounds before intact skin, cleaning the most contaminated areas first, using a radiation survey meter to monitor progress of decontamination, continuing decontamination until areas are below 2 to 3 times background radiation or there is no significant reduction between decontamination efforts

Specific Management

Symptomatic treatment is given in conditions like managing shock and hypoxia, relieving pain and anxiety, and giving sedatives to control seizures, antiemetics to control vomiting, and anti diarrhoeal agents for diarrhoea. There is no specific treatment for the cerebrovascular syndrome. The GI syndrome is treated with aggressive fluid resuscitation and electrolyte replacement. Management of the hematopoietic syndrome is similar to that of bone marrow hypoplasia and pancytopenia of any cause. Cytokines may be helpful.

Chapter 8

Plant Toxicology

☆ *Rajeev Ranjan and Naveen Kumar*

The toxic plant is one which causes biochemical or physiological changes when consumed by livestock. The effects of toxic plants may vary from mild sickness to death depends on type of toxin and amount that consumed by animals. Plants contain a large number of biologically active toxins. These toxins present naturally in plants as they are usually secondary metabolites produced by plants to evolve multiple defense mechanisms by which they are able to cope with their stress.

The identification of toxic plants is difficult, since toxic plants do not appear distinct from their nontoxic counterparts. Toxic principle may contain either in seed, root, leaf, stalk and fruit or throughout the whole plant. In others they are concentrated in one or more parts. The amount of toxin and degree of toxicity depends on the location, climatic factors, soil types, season, fertilization, plant variety and age. Some toxic plants have unpleasant tastes. Sometimes animals will often eat such plants only when other suitable feedstuffs are unavailable. However, some poisonous plants are very palatable if eaten in large quantity, it can cause serious problems.

Plant toxins may enter into the body by different route such as inhalation, ingestion or by direct contact. The action is mainly dependent on their phytoconstituents or active principle like alkaloids, glycosides, proteins, tannins, terpenes *etc.* The doses of exposure of these substances are the most important factor. Some of these have been found to be extremely useful for treating various diseases (*e.g.* digitoxin, vincristine, colchicines, *etc.*). But it may cause extremely toxicity at above the therapeutic dose. However, some plant constituents produce adverse effects following exposure. There are thousands of plants present in the environment but few plants cause acute and life-threatening illnesses after ingestion.

The diagnosis of plant poisonings is very difficult because many plants produce non-specific clinical signs that must be differentiated from other disease conditions. In addition, death due to plant toxic often does not show any characteristic post mortem lesions. The best way to diagnose the plant poisoning is the presence of a toxic plant in the animal's body as plants have been chewed and finding plant fragments in vomitus or gastrointestinal tract. However, some laboratory tests are available to detect plant toxins.

Plants have wide range of phytochemical substances. Although few plant phytochemicals produce harmful effects after exposure. On the basis of chemical nature, phytochemicals broadly classified into following groups. Within each group, there is remarkable chemical heterogeneity.

1. Alkaloids
2. Glycosides
3. Terpenes
4. Oxalates
5. Phenolics
6. Proteinaceous
7. Resins

1. Alkaloids

In pure form most alkaloids are colourless, nonvolatile, crystalline solids and bitter in taste. The chemical structures of alkaloids are extremely variable. Generally, alkaloids are nitrogen containing complex organic compounds. They are insoluble in water but readily soluble in alcohol. Alkaloid names generally end in the suffix- "ine", a reference to their chemical classification as amines. Alkaloids are found primarily in plants and are common in certain families of plants like Ranunculaceae (*e.g.*, buttercups) and Solanaceae (*e.g.*, nightshades) are prominent alkaloid-containing families of plants.

2. Glycoside

It is a molecule in which sugar group is attached to a non-sugar (aglycone or genin) part via a glycosidic bond. They are mostly soluble in alcohol but less soluble in water and insoluble in ether. In many plants, glycoside is stored in an inactive form. After hydrolysis, glycoside gets activated and sugar part to be broken off, making them available for use. Glycosides can be classified by the glycone, by the type of glycosidic bond, and by the aglycone. Classification of glycoside on the basis of chemical nature of the aglycone is the most relevant in toxicology. Common glycoside includes cyanogenic, cardiac, anthraquinone and coumarin.

3. Terpenes

Terpenes are a class of organic compounds, produced by a variety of plants. Terpene is a five-carbon isoprene unit. They are mostly hydro-carbons. The difference between terpenes and terpenoids is that terpenes are hydrocarbons, whereas terpenoids contain additional functional groups. Based on the number of the isoprene units contained inside the molecule, terpenes can be divided into monoterpene, sesquiterpene, diterpene, *etc.* Most of the terpenes are insoluble in water but soluble in ethanol, chloroform and diethyl ether.

4. Oxalates

They are present in many plants. Oxalic acid is a dicarboxylic acid. It is probably the strongest organic acid in plants. Oxalate occurs in many plants, where it is synthesized by the incomplete oxidation of carbohydrates. Soluble oxalate is an anti-nutrient in forage plants. It exerts its effects by binding with dietary calcium (Ca) or magnesium (Mg) to form insoluble Ca or Mg oxalate, which may lead to low serum Ca or Mg levels as well as renal failure because of precipitation of these salts in the kidneys. The salt of sodium (Na), potassium (K) and magnesium (Mg) oxalates is less soluble in water as compared to oxalic acid. High levels of oxalate in pasture plants were considered as a major factor in urolith formation in grazing animals.

5. Phenolics

Phenolics or phenols are made of a hydroxyl group bonded to an aromatic hydrocarbon. Phenolic compounds are classified as simple phenols or polyphenols based on the number of phenol units in the molecule.

Phenolic, like furanocoumarins, is non-toxic until activated by light. Furanocoumarin is responsible for the phytophotodermatitis seen in exposure to the juices of the wild parsnip and the giant hogweed. It blocks the transcription and repair of DNA.

6. Resins

Resins are phenolic compound and produced by oxidation and polymerization of volatile oils. Resins exude or ooze out from plant tissues through resin duct or giving incision on a particular area of the plants and tend to harden on exposure to air. They are insoluble in water but are soluble in ordinary solvents like alcohol, ether and turpentine. They are brittle, amorphous, transparent or semi-transparent. With the exception of lac, which is produced by the lac insect (*Kerria lacca*), all other natural resins are of plant origin.

7. Protenaceous Compound

There are number of protein toxins produced by plants enter into animal body or cells and inhibit protein synthesis enzymatically and producing severe toxic effect in multiple organ systems. Some examples of poisonous proteins include ricin (castor plant) and abrin (rosary pea).

Classification of Toxic Plants Based on Chemical Nature of their Active Constituents

Chemical Groups		Name of Plants	Active Principle
Alkaloids	Tropane	*Atropa belladonna, Datura stramonium, Hyoscyamus niger*	Atropine
	Pyrrolizidine	*Senecio aureus, Crotalaria spectabilis, Heliotropium indicum*	Retronecine
	Phenylamine	*Ephedra vulgaris, Ephedra sinica*	Ephedrine
	Diterpenoid	*Aconitum japonicum, Aconitum laciniatum*	Aconite
	Steroidal	*Solanum americanum*	Solanidine
	Pyrrolidine	*Nicotiana tabacum*	Nicotine
	Purine	*Coffea arabica*	Caffein
	Quinolone	*Cinchona officinalis*	Quinine
	Isoquinolone	*Papaver somniferum*	Morphine
	Indole	*Strychnous nuxvomica*	Strychnine
	Piperidine	*Conium maculatum*	Coniine, Conhydrine, Coniceine
Glycoside	Cynogenic	*Linum usitatissimum, Holcus lanatus, Trifolium repens*	Linamarin
		Sorghum vulgare, Sorghum sudanense	Dhurin
		Prunus amygdalus, Prunus avium	Amygdaline
		Strophantus gratus	Strophanthin
	Cardiac	*Digitalis purpurea, Nerium oleander*	Digitoxin
		Urgenia maritime	Proscillaridin A
	Anthraquinone	*Cassia fistula, Rheum undulatum*	Rhein
	Coumarin	*Aesculus californica*	Esculin/Aesculin
	Monoterpene	*Anamirta cocculus*	Picrotoxin
Terpenes	Sesquiterpenes	*Helenium microcephalum*	Helenalin
	Diterpenes	*Aconitum napellus*	Aconitine
	Triterpenes	*Lanatana camara*	Lantadenes
Protenaceous compound	Toxalbumin	*Abrus precatorius*	Abrin
		Ricinus communis	Ricin
	Polypeptide	*Amanita phalloides*	Amatoxin
	Amines	*Sativus odoratus*	Aminotryptaline
		Mimosa pudica	Miomosine
		Leucaena leucocephala	Mimosine
		Canavalia ensiformis	Canavanine

Chemical Groups	Name of Plants	Active Principle
	Brassia hyssopifolia	Oxalates
Oxalates	*Beta vulgaris*	
	Halogeton glomeratus	
	Pennisetum clandestinum	
	Rheum rhaponticum	
	Rumex crispus	
	Sarcobatus vermiculatus	
Phenolics	*Pastinaca sativa*	Furocoumarin
	Dictamnus albus	
	Heracleum mantegazzianum	
Resin	*Cannabis sativa*	Tetrahydrocannabinol
	Hypericum perforatum	Hypericin

Chapter 9

Plant Toxicity

Lantana

☆ *Rajeev Ranjan and T.J. Sheikh*

Scientific Name

Lantana camara L.

Common Names

Wild Sage, Bunch Berry, Baraphulnoo, Sleeper Weed, Panchful booty *etc.*

Lantana camara is one of the most commonly known poisonous weed, has diverse and broad geographic distribution. It had been introduced in India as an ornamental plant. Its exposure is the major cause of poisoning among livestock during droughts. It is a noxious weed, has established in many regions of the world. They can propagate in adverse soil and weather condition like wastelands, rain forests, riparian zones, urban areas, wetlands and forests recovering from fire. The species also thrive well in disturbed areas which include roadside, railways' tracks and canals. This plant produces hepatotoxicity, intrahepatic cholestasis and photosensitization in most of the animals due to presence of phytotoxin present in this plant.

Lantana camara is a low, erect, vigorous shrub. The leaf is ovate in shape and arranged in opposite pairs. Leaves are bright green, rough, finely hairy with serrate margins and emit pungent odour when crushed. The stem is woody, square in cross section and hairy when young. It is often non thorny with re-curved prickles. Flower heads contain 20-40 flowers; the colour varies from white, yellow to orange pink, purple and red depending on the location and plant maturity. Flowering occurs between August and March or all year round if adequate moisture and light are available. The fruit is a greenish blue-black colour, drupaceous, shining, with two nutlets.

Chemical Nature of Toxins

The most important toxic principle present in lantana is lantadene, a pentacyclic triterpenoid present in this weed. The major lantadenes are lantadene- A, B, C and D which have a common core structure of 22-hydroxy-oleanonic acid. Lantadenes are pentacyclic triterpenes and often led to hepatotoxicity, photosensitization and jaundice. Other toxic principles present in lantana are pentacyclic triterpene acids like Icterogenin, Dihydrolantadene A and reduced lantadene.

Transfer of lantana toxins to milk, placenta, or to the offspring has not been reported, but some teratological effects has been seen in rats. Lantadenes are also having effects on reproductive system, it interfere with the sperm count, daily sperm production and sperm morphology. The LD_{50} value of lantadene in sheep is 1-3 mg/kg body weight, when administered by intravenous route, while the LD_{50} value is 60 mg/kg body weight when administered by oral route, because of slow absorption.

The toxic effects of this plant are evident both in ruminants as well as in non-ruminants. Among ruminants cattle, buffalo and sheep are highly susceptible, while goats are little resistant to lantadene toxicity.

Mechanism of Toxicity

In lantana poisoning, the ruminal contents become more toxic with the passage of time due to the contents becoming more liquid and thus enhancing absorption. Toxin absorbed from all part of gastrointestinal tract (GIT) but maximum absorption occurs in small intestine. The toxin is transported to the liver mainly via portal blood. The absorbed toxins interact with biomolecules in hepatocytes and sequence of biochemical events leading to lantana toxicity. Toxin causes paralysis of gall bladder and closure of bile canaliculi leading to decrease bile flow. Cholestasis leads to regurgitation of bile, which causes marked increase in the levels of bilirubin and phylloerythrin (biodegradation product of chlorophyll) in blood circulation. Both bilirubin and phylloerythrin undergoes photochemical reaction on exposure to light which causes photosensitization and associate skin lesion.

This photochemical reaction cause excess production of free radical which damage the tissue. Tissue destruction causes release of histamine from the mast cells that initiates local inflammatory reaction and produces erythma, oedema, vesicles, pruritis, necrosis, local cell death or sloughing of the tissue *etc.* The sequel of ingestion of lantana plant is as shown in Figure 9.1.

Clinical Sign and Symptoms

Clinical signs of lantana poisoning depend on the amount and type of lantana consumed and the intensity of sunlight to which the animals have been exposed.

(i) Phylloerythrin, a degradation product of chlorophyll formed by the action of the GIT microorganisms get accumulated in the liver leads to photosensitization. This type of photosensitization is also called as hepatogenous photosensitization, which occurs due to the impaired hepatobiliary excretion.

(ii) Photosensitive animals are photophobic (photosensitisation) when exposed to sunlight.

(iii) Animals feel discomfort and scratches or rubs lightly pigmented areas of skin.

(iv) Reddening and inflammation of un-pigmented skin like muzzle, ears, eyelids and feet.

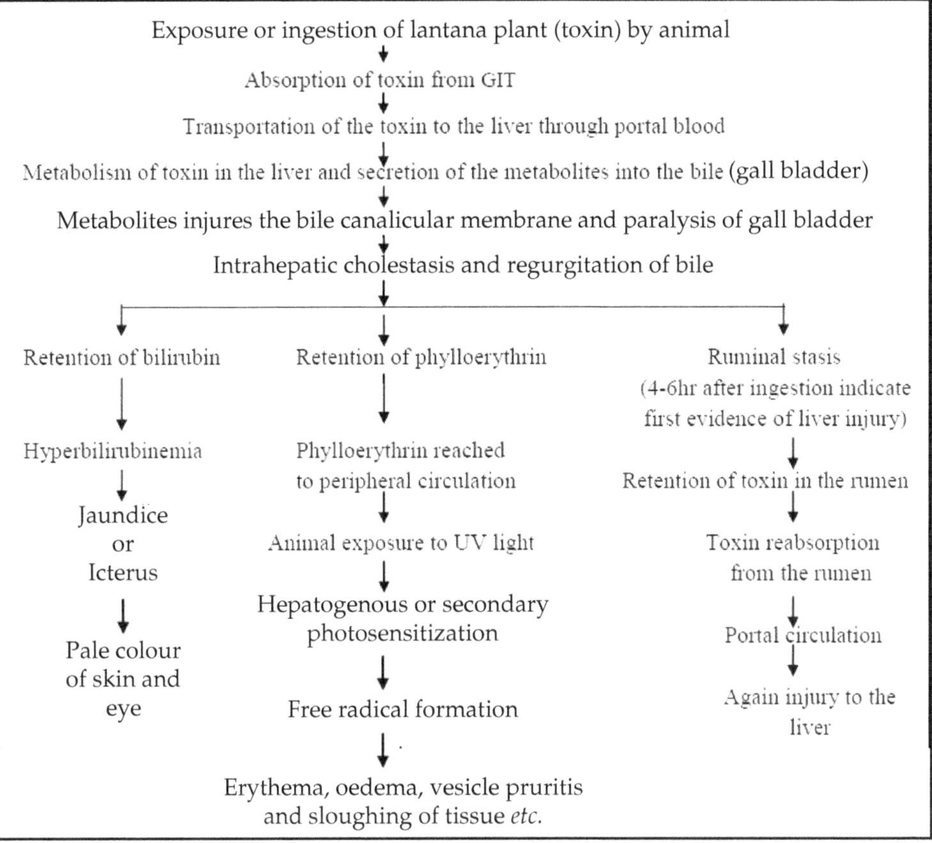

Figure 9.1

(v) Muzzle may become inflamed, moist, ulcerated and very painful (pink nose) and slough.

(vi) Yellow discolouration (due to jaundice) of the sclera of eye, conjunctiva, gums, skin of the nose and mouth and vulvar or vaginal mucous membranes.

(vii) Reddening and discharge from the eyes (conjunctivitis).

(viii) Ulceration of the tip and under surface of the tongue (if unpigmented). In chronic cases, the affected skin may slough leaving raw ulcerated surfaces.

(ix) Severely affected animals may suffer from constipation most commonly or diarrhoea for short period with strong-smelling black fluid faeces.

(x) Parenchymal cells lying to the periphery of the liver are damaged. Hepatocellular damage causes intrahepatic cholestasis along with the inhibition of bile secretions, accumulation of bilirubin and ultimately jaundice.

(xi) Further, animal exhibits depression, rumen stasis, loss of appetite, frequent urination and dehydration. Animal may succumb within 2 day to 3weeks.

Post-mortem Examination

(a) Mucus membranes: Pale

(b) Tissue: Yellowish discoloration.

(c) Faeces: Hard, dry, mucus-covered faecal masses in large intestine.

(d) Rumen: Dry undigested plant material in the rumen.

(e) Liver: Swollen, fragile, pale yellow, mottled with rounded edges.

(f) Kidneys: Swollen, pale and yellowish brown.

(g) Gall bladder: 3-4 times enlarged with dark opaque and viscous contents.

Histopathological/Biochemical Examination

☆ Haematological examination reveals increase in blood clotting time and hematocrit values but decrease in erythrocyte sedimentation rate.

☆ Biochemical examination reveal that there is an increase in phylloerythrin level, increase in serum bilirubin, AST, ALP, serum total protein, serum albumin and serum globulin and decrease in albumin/globulin ratio.

☆ Histopathological examination reveals that degeneration of the periportal parenchymal cells, distended bile canaliculi, fatty degeneration, portal fibrosis, hyperplasia of bile ducts and edema of gall bladder walls.

☆ In chronic cases the myofibroblasts produce type 1 collagen which leads to fibrous tissue formation, may induce chronic liver fibrosis.

Diagnosis

Diagnosis is based on history, clinical sign, biochemical examination, post-mortem examination and histopathological findings.

Treatment

Specific treatment for lantana toxicity is not available. The symptomatic and supportive therapy gives desired response.

i. Provide oral electrolytes or intravenous fluids and encouraging the animal to eat.

ii. Administration of activated charcoal or bentonite (cheaper than the charcoal) 5 gram/kg body weight with electrolyte (in stomach) tube within 24 h, which reduces the absorption of toxin.

iii. Other supportive therapy include:

  ☆ Oral administration of liver tonics.

  ☆ Administration of Vitamin B-complex.

  ☆ Corticosteroid should be administered.

  ☆ NSAIDs should be administered.

☆ H$_1$ antihistsminics should be used.

☆ Administration of antibiotics will help to prevent secondary infection.

iv. Bacterial strains like *Pseudomonas picketii, Alcaligenes faecalis* and *Alcaligenes odorans* can be used which degrades the lantadenes.

v. Rumenotomy can be done to evacuate the toxic contents from GI tract.

Prevention

The preventive measures are more effective than curative measures to reduce the harmful effects of this notorious weed. There are different ways by which lantana propagation can be prevented. It is the cost effective way to prevent our animals from being poisoned by lantana.

☆ Prevent exposure of the animals to the noxious weed.

☆ Keep your land lantana free by weed control measurement.

☆ Regular burning will reduce the number of plants.

☆ Biological control of plants by predator moths, flea beetles and seed flies is another tool to reduce the number of plants.

☆ Never put new stock in areas where lantana is present.

☆ Move the intoxicated animals away from light.

☆ Keep the animals in a well shaded area, away from the direct sun light.

☆ Educate and communicate people regarding the harmful effects of this noxious weed.

☆ Collaboration with government agencies, so that outline can be made to prevent the spread of lantana.

☆ The international standards for trading partner countries in a well targeted form must be implemented.

Bracken Fern

☆ *Nrip Kishore Pankaj*

Scientific Name

Pteridium aquilinum

Common Name

Bracken fern

Bracken fern is widespread all over the world (except the extreme climatic conditions) and grows in semi shaded areas with moderate moisture and well-drained soil especially in acidic forest soils, warm dark areas of woods, and road sides. They grow and propagate by rhizome and can form dense vegetation. *Equisetum spp.* (horsetail) is found in wet areas, usually near water body. It can grows up to 150 cm in height, has fronds, stems and rhizomes. Rhizomes are most toxic part of bracken fern. Bracken fern hay retains toxicity. In Some part of the world such as such as Japan, Brazil, Canada, and China people consume bracken crosiers as a delicacy and a source of nutrients such as protein, carbohydrates, fat, vitamins, carotenoids, and trace minerals. Sheep are generally less prone to bracken fern toxicity as compared to cattle.

Toxic Principles

Major toxic principles in bracken fern are Ptaquiloside and Thiaminase. Ptaquiloside is a **terpenoid** glucoside, is the major carcinogen of bracken, also induce bone marrow suppression and anemia in ruminants, especially sheep and cattle therefore also called aplastic anemia factor.

1. Ptaquiloside

The risk of bracken fern exposure among livestock depends upon the hunger and availability of green fodder. Hungry cattle may consume large amounts of available green bracken fern when other healthy fodder is unavailable. However, regular consumption of small amounts of bracken over years together leads to tumour of urinary tract or digestive tract. The most common syndrome is aplastic anemia in cattle, which is associated with acute toxicity. Bracken fern causes fibrosarcoma of the mandible in sheep and tumours of the upper alimentary tract in cattle. Hematuria factor found in bracken fern is responsible for enzootic hematuria.

Toxicosis of bracken fern amount to various health concerns, depends upon age of the animal, duration and rate of consumption and toxin content in the plant, which depends upon climatic condition. Toxidrome of bracken poisoning includes Bovine enzootic hematuria (BEH), characterised by chronic haemorrhage in the urinary bladder or tumors in the bladder wall among affected cattle.

Mechanism of Toxicity

Ptaquiloside is the compound in bracken fern, assumed to cause death of precursor cells in the bone marrow and induce genesis of tumor in the urinary tract. The ileum and the urine of herbivores are alkaline. Under weakly alkaline conditions both ptaquiloside and its aglycone ptaquilosin are converted into the unstable dienone, is regarded as the ultimate carcinogen. Ptaquilosin is strongly electrophilic and reacts readily with amino acids, nucleosides and nucleotides under mild conditions, forming covalent adducts with DNA and results in to break in DNA strands.

In the field, cattle and sometimes sheep grazing on bracken fern develop tumours, most frequently in the ileum and urinary bladder. Ptaquiloside has been found in the milk of cows feeding on bracken fern. Regular bracken exposure leads in to a chronic haematuria in cattle characterised by haemorrhages (Bovine enzootic haematuria (BEH) and tumour in the urinary bladder.

Clinical Signs and Symptoms

The toxicity sign appears on feeding 3 to 4 kg fresh bracken for over three months such as:

   i. Suppression of bone marrow activity or aplastic anemia due to consumption of young fronds.
   ii. Leukopenia with the disappearance of all WBC components except lymphocytes.
   iii. Prolongation of bleeding time.
   iv. Haemorrhages in anterior chamber of the eyes, over mucous membranes (vulva, mouth and conjunctiva) and skin leads to blood-stained sweating in cattle and sheep.
   v. Acute rises of body temperature to 40.5– 41.0 °C.
   vi. The faeces may contain fresh and digested blood.
   vii. Enzootic hematuria: frequent loss of blood via hemorrhages and tumors of the urinary bladder.
   viii. Reduction in the level of Ca, P and thiamine.
   ix. Lethargy, loss of appetite, elevated heart rate, weakness and death.

In sheep, ptaquiloside induces stenosis of vessels supplying retina leading to progressive retinal atrophy among animals over 18 months of age. The retinal atrophy leads to increased reflectance of *Tapetum lucidum,* noticed in semi dark ambience termed as Bright blindness. The affected sheep exhibit blindness, high-stepping gait and dilated pupils with poor light reflex.

Clinical Pathology

Thromobocytopenia may be marked in asymptomatic herd mates that have not yet become noticeably ill. Blood-loss anemia and blood in the urine are expected with chronic enzootic hematuria.

Post-mortem Finding

1. Neoplasm of upper digestive tract along with neo-plastic nodule and sub-epithelial haemorrhages alternating with ulcerative lesions in urinary bladder.

2. Haemorrhages along with necrosis in kidney and presence of calculi in the renal tubules.

3. Liver exhibits bile duct hyperplasia and fibrous tissue proliferation

4. Bone marrow suppression primarily affects thrombocyte and granulocyte production

5. Necropsy of the cattle died of aplastic anemia exhibit numerous points of small and large haemorrhages in thoracic pleura, epicardium, laryngeal mucosa, visceral serosa, gall bladder and urinary bladder lining. Squamous cell carcinoma is observed in the upper digestive tract. Tumors associated with enzootic hematuria may be benign or malignant. Bladder tumours are most common in cattle, but may be in the ureters and renal pelves as well.

Treatment

Blood or platelet transfusion might be useful in cattle with aplastic anemia. Antibiotics may prevent secondary infections.

Prognosis

The mortality rate in cattle with bone marrow failure is nearly 100 per cent. A rising thrombocyte count suggests some hope of recovery. Usually the chances of recovery among bracken fern exposed animals are bleak.

2. Thiaminase

Thiaminase are enzmyes found in a bracken fern, horsetails (*Equisetum arvense*) and viscera of certain fish. Thiaminase splits thiamine (Vitamin B_1 which play important role in energy metabolism) and render it inactive. Their ingestion can spell trouble to livestock and humans.

Ruminants

Ruminants are relatively resistant to thiamine deficiency owing to its synthesis by ruminal microbes. However, ingestion of thiaminases by cattle may leads to polioencephalomalacia. Growing cattle and sheep, fed with high-grain diets are more vulnerable to toxicity. Grains dominant ration can facilitate propagation of thiaminase producing bacteria in the rumen such as *Clostridium sporogenes* and *Bascillus.* These lead to production of enough thiaminase to induce thiamine deficiency.

Thiamine deficiency in ruminants gets manifested as polioencephalomalacia, characterized by disorientation, wandering, blindness and opishotonus. The brain of infected animals becomes inflamed and edematous. Ruminants also show symptoms as seen in other animals.

Non-ruminant

Thiamine pyrophosphate is an obligate cofactor in several reactions in carbohydrate metabolism. Both *P. aquilinum* and *Equisetum arvense* also contains thiaminase, which destroys dietary thiamine (in to inactive components *i.e.* thiazole and pyrimidine) before its absorption in the gut. Thiamine is required for the synthesis of acetyl coenzyme A from pyruvate, and for conversion of α-ketoglutarate in to succinyl coenzyme-A in Kerbs' cycle. This compromises availability of thiamine, thus compromises the intermediary energy metabolism. This declines cellular stores of adenosine triphosphate (ATP) and lead to surge of pyruvate concentration in the peripheral blood. Further, it impairs the neuronal (CNS) functions, manifested as depression and polioencephalomalacia observed in horses and pigs.

Clinical Signs

Bracken fern toxicity in non ruminant animals are similar to the deficiency of thiamine. The symptoms may include lethargy, anorexia, weight loss and emaciation followed by ataxia, in coordination and staggering gait (bracken stagger) among mules and horses. The animals progressively get uncoordinated, exhibit wider stance, and develops posterior paralysis and fail to rise on feet. The heart rate becomes weak and fast and even slight exercise leads to exhaustion. The animals may exhibit muscle fasciculation (on exercise) and spasm, progress to terminal opisthotonus, convulsions, and death. Other signs include elevated pyruvate concentration in blood, decline in blood thiamine level and cardiac arrythymia. Horse may exhibit colic, hemoglobinurea, anemia, pyrexia, tachycardia and may succumb in 2-10 days if left untreated.

Rabbits exposed to bracken fern exhibit progressive anaemia, leukopenia, lymphopenia and relative heterophilia along with elevated activity of serum transaminase (SGPT), alkaline phosphatase (ALP), urea and creatinine. The visceral organs exhibit vascular changes, vacuolar degenerations of the hepatocytes, intestine remains in hyper-secretary mode and presence of casts in renal tubules.

Birds exhibit retraction of the head (opisthotonus) referred to as "star-gazing".

As such thiamine deficiency does not result in any specific changes. No specific gross lesions are found at necropsy. In addition to the circumstances, history and risk of bracken fern consumption, response to therapy with thiamine point to the diagnosis. Else blood thiamine assay can confirm the diagnosis. In the presence of thiaminase, blood thiamine levels in horses can reduce from a normal level 80-100 mg/L to 25-30 µg/L and in contrast, the pyruvate level gets elevated from 20mg/L normal to 85mg/L. The episodes of acute haemorrhage should be differentiated from babesiosis, sweet clover poisoning and anthrax.

Treatment

Non-ruminants

Thiamine @5mg/Kg. body weight *via* intravenous route three times a day initially followed by intramuscular route, later orally for few weeks. However, thiamine administered @100 to 200 mg twice on the first day and then daily for few weeks helps to recover from the bracken fern toxicity.

Ruminants

The animal should be debarred from any further exposure to the bracken fern and horse tail plants. As such there are no specific antidote available, needs to be treated symptomatically. Although of limited value, DL-Batyl alcohol @ 1gm/10ml of olive oil can be used for 4-5 days through subcutaneous route. Transfusion of healthy blood or platelets may be of some help. Antibiotics may be opted to control secondary bacterial infection.

Prognosis

Early cases respond well to the treatment and prognosis is good. If the animal has exhibited advanced signs, the prognosis is poor.

Diagnosis

It depends upon prevalence of bracken fern in the area/pasture, circumstantial evidence and history of exposure over months rightly correlating clinical signs and symptoms in support to its diagnosis.

Prevention and Control

The chances of exposure of bracken fern in the pasture should be reduced by management practices. The risk is greatest in the weather when young, tender fronds propagate and suitable forage is limited. The animals at the risk of exposure may also be considered for vaccination against bovine papillomavirus, may reduce the incidence of bracken fern–induced tumours.

Castor Bean

☆ *Nrip Kishore Pankaj and Shahid Prawez*

Scientific Name

Ricinus communis L.

Common Names

Arandi, castor.

The toxicity of castor seeds has been recognized since ancient times. It has been mentioned in Egyptian and Greek literature including Susruta Ayurveda. The castor oil plant (*Ricinus communis L.*), belongs to family Euphorbiaceae. This plant is highly toxic due to its active principle ricin. Ricin is also known as hemaglutinin or toxalbumin. It is one of the most toxic glycoprotein (or lectin), with affinity for sugar molecules. The endosperm of castor seeds is rich in ricin, however it is present in lower amounts in the rest of the plant like leaves and stem. All animals (livestock and pets) are vulnerable to ricin.

Ricinus communis L. is an oil seed plant contains 50 per cent of its seed's dry weight as oil. Its oil is used for cosmetics and industrial purposes. India is one of the major contributors of the world's castor oil. The major constituent of castor oil is ricinoleic acid along with little amount of various compounds *i.e.* dihydroxystearic acid, linoleic acid, oleic acid, stearic acids *etc.* Castor oil is commonly used in various industries of resin and plastic, pharmaceuticals as cosmetics and laxative, textile and leather industries *etc.* The ricin is water soluble, heat labile toxalbumin, doesn't get extracted in the oil fraction therefore remains in the seed cake only. Ricin is classified as a Category B agent by the US Centers for Disease Control and Prevention (CDC). Ricin is also monitored as a Schedule 1 agent under the Chemical Weapons Convention.

Toxic Principle

The castor seeds contain toxic glycoproteins (ricin), ricinoleic acid (12-hydroxyoleic acid) and the alkaloid ricinine. Ricinine is an indicator of the presence of material from castor beans in press cakes in feeding stuffs for animals. Purified ricin, which exists as a white powder, is stable over a wide pH range when dissolved in water, and inactivation requires heating at 80°C for an hour. Solid forms of ricin would require either higher temperatures or extended duration of heating to ensure inactivation. Various vegetable oil has direct laxative effect due to its irritating properties on the small intestine. Castor oil is hydrolyzed by lipase in the small intestine and form sodium and potassium salts which act as soaps, produces irritation thereby laxation. Ricinoleic acid is the one of the most potent compound that produces rapid and complete colonic emptying. This clinical effect is seen 4–8 h after administration of castor oil in small animals, and 12–18 h post dosing in large animals. Animals treated with castor oil should be fed moist, bulky material afterward.

Mechanism of Toxicity

Castor beans contain two lectins *i.e.* ricin I and ricin II, in which later one is more toxic. Ricin is a potent cell toxin, a type II ribosomal inhibitory protein (RIP II).

Ricin II is composed of A and B amino acid chains, of approximately 30 kDa each linked by a disulfide bond. Mammalian cells do contain a large number of glycoproteins and glycolipids with galactose residues that are available for the B chain of ricin to attach. The B chain of the ricin molecules is a sugar binding protein, binds to galactoside-containing proteins on the cell surface, facilitate internalization *i.e.* endocytosis of the toxin.

Ultimately, the A chain is translocated from cytosol to the endoplasmic reticulum, depurinates 28S ribosomal ribonucleic acid (rRNA) by the removal of a specific adenine residue. Thus, protein synthesis is interfered, leads to cell death. Ricin also reduces Ca^{++} uptake by sarcoplasmic reticulum and enhance Na^{+}-Ca^{++} exchange thus affects calcium homeostasis in the cardiovascular system.

In addition to protein synthesis inhibition, other mechanisms of toxicity include apoptosis, magnesium and calcium imbalances, cytokine release, acute phase reactions, and oxidative stress in the liver. Poisoning may happen in dogs, poultry, wild fowl, pigs, horses, sheep, and goats.

Clinical Signs and Symptoms

Ruminants

The ricin toxicity is dose dependent among cattle. Raw castor seed contains 55 to 58 gm/kg ricin, is toxic. Outbreaks of ricin poisoning in cattle fed rations contaminated with castor bean husks have been described. The symptoms in dairy cows include a fall in milk yield followed by depression, inappetence and severe diarrhoea. The ricin poisoning is often fatal, and if the exposed animals survived, needs over a week to recover. Intense inflammation with sloughing of mucous membranes of abomasum and intestines along with petechiae of the heart has been observed in post mortem examination.

In sheep, a dose dependent acute tubular necrosis in kidney has been found along with elevated alanine aminotransferase, aspartate aminotransferase levels, lymphocytosis, neutrophilia, histo-morphological alterations in liver, intestine, spleen and lymph nodes. The dose of ricin @ 1.4 and 2.8 mg/kg body weight per day in sheep develops toxicity by symptoms like dark brown urine and faeces and exhibit congested kidney, intestinal mucous membrane along with thick, mucous exudates on post mortem examination.

Among poultry, approximately 10 g/kg body weight per day of castor beans leads to reduction feed intake and weight gain followed by high mortality in growing chicks. A single dose of approximately 1 g/kg body weight of castor bean husk leads to poisoning in pullets. In ducks lethal dose is approximately 0.7-1.2 g castor beans per kg body weight. The common symptoms are dullness, drooping wings, ruffled feathers and greyish-coloured wattles and combs. The clinical signs resemble those of botulism, except for mucoid, blood-tinged excreta. The commonest lesions were severe fatty change in the liver, widely distributed internal petechial haemorrhages or eccymoses, and catarrhal enteritis.

Ricin is approximately 1000-fold more toxic following parenteral administration or inhalation, than by the oral route. Oral LD_{50} values in rats and mice were 20 to 30 mg/kg body weight, and the corresponding intra peritoneal LD_{50} value for mice is 22 μg/kg body weight. The LD_{50} in dogs is 1-1.75 μg/kg body weight when injected. Symptoms often develop within 6 hours of castor bean ingestion in dogs. Castor bean toxicosis in animals often happens several hours after ingestion of the beans. Dogs show symptoms within 1.5 to 6 days duration in dogs. The most hazardous routes of ricin exposure are inhalation and injection. Intramuscular injection induces severe localized pain and necrosis of regional lymph nodes and muscles with moderate systemic signs. Features of toxicity mainly reflect damage to cells of the reticuloendothelial system, with fluid and protein loss, bleeding, oedema and impaired cellular defense against endogenous toxins.

The lethal dose by inhalation (breathing in solid or liquid particles) and injection (into muscle or vein) in human is approximately 5-10 micrograms/kg of body weight.

Diagnosis

Techniques like enzyme-linked immunosorbent assays (ELISA) do exist for the identification of ricin in tissue sections, body fluids, environmental samples, and food. This method is also applied in human specimens with a lower limit of detection of 0.1 ng/mL (1.54 pmol/L).

Treatment

Ricin intoxicated subject is difficult to treat as it acts rapidly and irreversibly. Vaccination should be opted against probability of its use as weapon of biological warfare. Supportive and symptomatic care in all species is important.

Emesis can help within 2-3 hrs of animals' exposure. Activated charcoal @ 1 - 4 g/kg body weight orally and magnesium sulfate @ 250 mg/kg or 70 per cent sorbitol @ 3 ml/kg body weight *via* oral route can be helpful in removing ricin after its ingestion.

Kaolin-pectin or sucralfate @ 0.25 to 2 gm three times a day orally, helps by protecting the mucus membrane of intestine. Electrolyte therapy is important to correct hypotension considering daily needs as well as ricin toxicosis mediated fluid losses.

Bland diet should be opted regularly for several days after controlling vomition. If seizures happen due to ricin ingestions, diazepam @0.5 to 1 mg/kg body weight intravenously may be used. It needs repeated clinical biochemical evaluations, until enzyme levels are back to normal and resolve the issue. Antibiotics and lactulose @ 0.1 to 0.5 mg/kg body weight thrice a day orally can be helpful.

Prognosis

Absorption depends on mastication of seeds or else it is poorly absorbed and the mortality rate is low in all animals. Although, once the animal reflects signs of ricin toxicity, the prognosis is guarded.

Prevention

Ricin is heat labile, so if ricin containing feed is treated with heat before feeding, it can prevent incidence of toxicity. Castor beans should be kept out of reach from all animals including pets

Cyanogenic Plants

☆ *Nrip Kishore Pankaj and Dhirendra Kumar*

Hydrocyanic acid (cyanide or prussic acid) is one of the quickest acting toxin that affects mammals. Hydrogen cyanide was first isolated from Prussian blue (blue dye), is acidic therefore known as prussic acid. There are at least 2650 species of plants that produce cyanogenic glycosides along with hydrolytic enzyme (β-glycosidase) in separate compartment. These cyanogenic compounds are present in epidermal cells of the plant with highest levels in seeds, leaves, bark and twigs, lowest in fruit, while the enzymes that enable cyanide production are in the leaves. The cell structure of the plant is disrupted by a predator due to mastication. This facilitates the enzyme and substrate (cyanogenic glycosides) to react, with subsequent breakdown to sugar and a cyanohydrin. Cyanohydrin rapidly decomposes to free and volatile hydrogen cyanide (HCN), and an aldehyde or a ketone.

The glycosides, cyanohydrins and hydrogen cyanide are collectively known as cyanogens. This combination of cyanogenic glycoside and hydrolytic enzyme is the means by which cyanogenic plants are protected against predators. Seeds of members of the Rosaceae family including apple, cherry, peach and apricot do contain cyanogenic glycosides. A number of common plants used as fodder (*Sorghum vulgare* and its hybrids) may accumulate large quantities of cyanogenic compounds. Plants that contains cyanogens are summarized as under:

Plants	Botanical Name	Cyanogens
Sorghum	*Sorghum vulgare – leaves*	Dhurrin
Johnson grass	*Sorghum halepense*	Dhurrin
Sudan grass	*Sorghum sudanense*	Dhurrin
Bamboo	*Dendrocalamus giganteus*	Taxiphyllin
Linseed/Flax	*Linum usitatissimum*	Linamarin, linustatin, neolinustatin
Arrow grass	*Triclochin palustris, T. maritima*	Triglochinin, Taxiphillin
Clovers	*Trifolium spp*	Lotaustralin
Bitter Almond	*Prunus dulcis, Prunus amygdalus*	Amygdalin
Plum and Cherry	*Prunus spp.*	Amygdalin
Peaches	*Prunus persica – Kernel*	Amygdalin
Apricot	*Prunus armeniace – Kernel*	Amygdalin
Cassava	*Manihot esculenta*	Linamarin

Cyanide poisoning is a metabolic condition in livestock. Livestock owners need to understand the sources and causes as well as recognize the symptoms of cyanide poisoning, or else entire herds can be affected and can be devastating to their economic status. Animal owners should understand the risk factors and employ effective methods to prevent prussic acid poisoning

Factors affecting Toxicity

Ruminants usually detoxify 0.5gm of HCN/hr. Cyanogenic plants may contain variable amount of HCN ranging from few ppm to 8000 ppm of dry weight from the glycoside dhurrin in aerial parts of Sorghum (Burrows and Tyrl, 2001). Sudan grass having high content of HCN, used as fodder for livestock may be hazardous. Forage cyanide concentration over 200 ppm, deliver a dose of over 2 mg HCN/kg body weight and produce signs of acute toxicosis.

Ruminants are at the greatest risk of poisoning because they have the ability to consume large quantities of forage and other fibrous materials. However, other species such as pigs, horses, and house pets, can be at risk as well.

Cattle are most vulnerable because of microbial reduction of cyanogen; thereby liberation of HCN than non ruminants. Sheep are relatively resistant to cyanide toxicity than cattle due to the different set of enzyme in their fore-stomachs. Lower pH in the stomach of the monogastric like horse and pigs inactivates the vital β-glucosidase and lysase therefore are less susceptible.

Hydrocyanic acid is metabolized to formic acid and ammonium chloride to certain extent, thus relatively less toxic to non-ruminants.

Adverse climatic condition (hot/draught/icy cold), rain after hot and humid climate, physical damage to plant facilitates greater concentration of cyanogens in its tissues. Forage crops like Sorghum especially during pre-flowering stage contains high cyanogens level. Application of nitrate fertilizers and weedicide like **2, 4-Diphenoxyacetic acid** also facilitates cyanogens accumulation in the plants.

Toxicokinetics

The highest level of cyanide appears in the lungs and blood following oral exposure; simultaneously it does not get cumulated in the blood and tissues following chronic oral exposure. Cyanide is metabolized to thiocyanate in the body, with a plasma half life of 20 minutes to 1 hour. Thiocyanate gets eliminated mostly in urine although little CN^- is excreted via lungs yields bitter almond odour.

Mechanism of Toxicity

Fodder plants usually contains cyanogenic glycosides, β-glycosidase and hydroxynitrile lyase in different compartment. These enzymes come in contact with and hydrolyze the glycoside to hydroxynitrile and volatile HCN. The first step in this process yields a sugar/glycone and an aliphatic or aromatic α-hydroxynitrile aglycone, thereafter forms carbonyl compound such as an aldehyde or a ketone, (benzaldehyde) and HCN. Generally, hay loses most of the HCN prior to feeding.

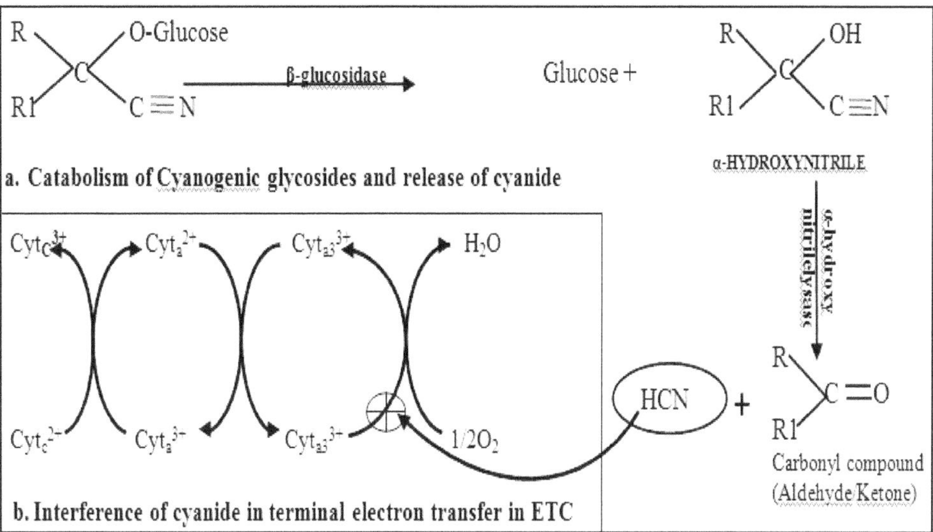

Cyanide affects practically all metalloenzymes, but its principal toxicity is derived owing to its (CN^-) high affinity to Fe^{3+} in cytochrome oxidase (in heme), inhibiting the functioning of the Electron Transport Chain (ETC). Thus, flux of electrons and the genesis of the H^+ ion gradient declines, leading to sudden severe decline in ATP production. This causes a decrease in the utilization of oxygen in the tissues leading to histotoxic anoxia. Cyanide causes an increase in blood glucose and lactic acid levels and a decrease in the ATP/ADP ratio indicating a shift from aerobic to anaerobic metabolism. Thus, oxyhemoglobin is carried in the venous blood, which is one biomarker of cyanide exposure. ATP is required for vital biological functions. The organ system having high oxygen demand (nervous tissue) require more ATP to let it maintain its function, therefore will suffer first.

Acute cyanide intoxication causes confusion, agitation, and disorientation because it impairs the nervous system and prevents normal cognition. Depending upon severity, if the nervous system is significantly impaired, soon death will follow due to respiratory and cardiac arrest.

In addition to binding to cytochrome c oxidase, cyanide inhibits catalase, peroxidase, hydroxocobalamin, phosphatase, tyrosinase, ascorbic acid oxidase, xanthine oxidase, and succinic dehydrogenase activities, which may also contribute to the signs of cyanide toxicity.

Toxidromes/Clinical Signs

Once cyanogenic plants are consumed by the animals, CN^- is rapidly transported *via* the blood throughout the body of the animal. When the animals' capacity to detoxify cyanide is superseded, oxygen utilization in the animal's body cells is impaired; animal suffocates and gasps for air. In per acute cases the animal/s may be dead within few minutes of exposure.

Acute Toxicity

In acute condition, toxidromes of poisoning commonly occur within 15–20 minutes following the consumption of cyanogenic plants. Death occurs within 1–2 hours in acute cases. In most of the cases, animals are found dead with no signs observed. The brain and heart are the first to be affected by lack of oxygen, and so the resulting clinical signs prior to death include: hyperpnoea, rapid, weak, irregular pulse (tachycardia), anxiety and restlessness followed by depression, stumbling/staggering, muscle tremors, moaning, dilated pupils, recumbency, bloat, and sometimes salivation and vomiting (ruminal regurgitation), excessive lacrimation, mydriasis, voiding of urine and faeces, tremor followed by fasciculation of muscles, terminal convulsions and death. Bright red mucous membranes finally turn cyanosed. A bitter almond-like odour can be noticed in the breath and ruminal content. However this odour is noticed by genetically determined individuals only.

Chronic Toxicity

Animal exposed to lower concentration of cyanide for longer duration may show symptoms like bradycardia, arrhythmia, T-wave abnormality, vomiting, increased blood urea nitrogen and histopathological changes of proximal tubular epithelium and glomeruli. Thyroid toxicity was also reported in intermediate-duration oral studies in rats and pigs.

Thyroid effects following cyanide exposure result from the interference of thiocyanate, a metabolite of cyanide, with iodine uptake and utilization in the thyroid gland. Reduced thyroid hormone levels, increasingly elevated levels of thyroid stimulating hormone and goiter are sequelae of chronic cyanide exposure in human in Africa.

Konzo is a neurological disease first time observed in younger people of Congo in 1938, later also found in other African countries due to consumption of cassava as a staple diet. It results in an irreversible spastic (stiff) paralysis of both legs.

Cyanide is detoxified by its conversion in to thiocyanate (SCN-) and dietary sulfur comes from protein. Cassava is a carbohydrate-rich food, very low in protein, thus it predisposes the chronic cyanide toxicity. It can be inferred that higher protein can be safe up to certain level.

Tropical Ataxic Neuropathy (TAN) is observed in older Nigerian people. It is believed to be due to feeding of poorly processed cassava with low protein intake. TAN is characterized by sensory neuropathy (unable to sense of touch), bilateral optic atrophy (loss of vision), bilateral deafness and sensory ataxia.

Diagnosis

Owing to acute onset hunger for air, bitter almond odour of breath and bright red mucus membrane along with types of fodder ingested by the animal can be helpful for tentative diagnosis. The samples for analysis are feed, ruminal/stomach content, heparinized blood, muscle and liver. The sample should be collected to its earliest following toxicosis/death, and placed in air tight poly bag, submitted in frozen state quickly to the laboratory for diagnosis. Care should be taken to avoid the loss of HCN being volatile therefore easily lost from the specimen. Cyanide in ruminal content over10 ppm may facilitate diagnosis.

Differential Diagnosis

In nitrate poisoning, the animal's tongue and eyes turn blue and blood becomes dark chocolate brown in colour. In contrast, prussic acid causes the animal's blood to turn a bright cherry red. In case of carbon mono oxide intoxication death is not quick as compared to HCN poisoning. Tissue and blood appear dark brown and emit H_2S in case of hydrogen sulphide toxicity. Ruminal content emit ammonia like odour in urea poisoning.

Treatment

Cyanide is very quick in producing the toxidrome owing to its rapid distribution; therefore it needs to be very quick and precise in dealing with recovery of cytochrome oxidase enzyme thereby reinstitution of cellular oxygenation. There are various approaches to treat cyanide poisoning in animals. Most common synchronous antidotal therapy is sodium nitrite followed by sodium thiosulfate.

Ruminants: Sodium nitrite is (20 per cent solution @20mg/kg body weight) **or** methylene blue (1 to 4 per cent solution, 2 to 3 g/225 kg. body weight) should be administered by slow intravenous route. Both should never be administered. Later sodium thiosulfate 20 per cent solution @ 500 mg/kg body weight intravenously should be administered, along with 25-30gm of sodium thiosulfate orally per large ruminant and 5-6 gm for each small ruminant.

Alternatively 1ml of 20 per cent sodium nitrite + 3ml of 20 per cent sodium thiosulfate *i.e.* 4ml of it per 45kg body weight IV can be administered. 1-4 per cent Methylene blue @2.5gm for 240kg body weight IV can be used in place of sodium nitrite.

Sodium nitrite (1-3 per cent) @25 mg/kg followed by sodium thiosulfate (25 per cent solution) @1.25gm/kg body weight should be given slowly *via* intravenous route in dogs and cats. In less severe cases of poisoning, sodium nitrite may not be required, only sodium thiosulfate and supportive measures may be sufficient. Half of the doses of sodium nitrite and sodium thiosulfate may be repeated in 30 minutes.

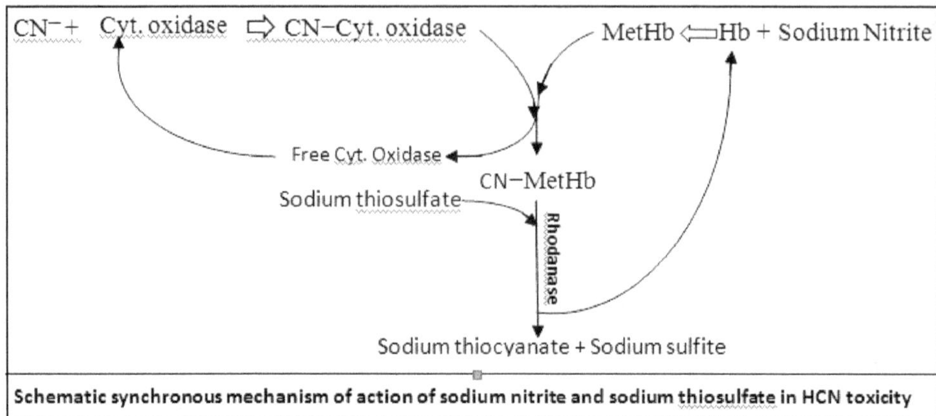

Schematic synchronous mechanism of action of sodium nitrite and sodium thiosulfate in HCN toxicity

Vinegar 3-4 L in 12-18 L cold water can be used in cattle to reduce microbial digestion.

Aquocobalamin (B_{12b}) or hydroxycobalamin (B_{12a}) forms stable complex with additional cyanide in blood circulation and gets eliminated *via* kidney therefore may be used at large dose (50 gm of hydroxycobalamin binds 1gm of CN⁻).

It is very important to manage the minimum gap between exposure of cyanogenic fodder and institution of treatment to observe the prognosis better. Usually if the animal survives for a day recovers well.

Prevention

There is a huge risk owing to quick and severe outcome of prussic acid poisoning and potentially devastating economically, therefore, preventive measure should be adopted. Immature stocks of Sorghum and sudan grasses should never be grazed when they are in preflowering state. New hybrid varieties of sudangrass and sorghum x sudangrass has lower prussic acid content may be considered as forage. However these hybrids too may accumulate enough HCN in inclement climatic condition. The animals should be fed some hay or so, before let the animals be left to the fresh pastures, as the hungry animals will be eating voraciously, will supervene the HCN level beyond its detoxification limits (500mg/hour). This will reduce the amount of prussic acid consumed and will buy more time for the animal to detoxify HCN at low level. The risk increases when only limited feed is available, resulting in animals being more attracted to nearby greens. The potentially toxic fodder should be processed, such as chopping, haying, or ensiling. This facilitates the HCN to volatilize, thus reducing it to acceptable levels in the feed.

Abrus

☆ *Nrip Kishore Pankaj and Rajinder Raina*

Scientific Name

Abrus precatorius

Common Names

Rosary bean, ratti, jequirity beans, gunja

The vine of *Abrus precatorius* is native to Southeast Asia. It is readily available, may pose public health problem. It has been classified as Category-B agent by the US Centers for Disease Control and Prevention (CDC). It is categorized as "Biological Select Agents or Toxins" by the US Department of Health and Human Services (HHS).

Abrin is the most toxic phytotoxin, closely related to ricin in its structure and properties, obtained from *Abrus precatorius*, a tropical ornamental plant. To name few of its many names are rosary bean, ratti, jequirity beans, gunja *etc.* Its seeds are very attractive and usually scarlet (red and black) colour and of 3 × 8mm in size. It had been used in weighing precious metal. It has also been used in malicious toxicity as needle (*sui*) toxicity in animals.

Mechanism of Toxicity

Abrin was first isolated as galactose-binding lectins. It belongs to the group of type-2 ribosome-inactivating proteins (RIPs). Abrin is heterodimeric glycoproteins composed of two polypeptides chain *i.e.* A-chain (approx. 30 kDa) and B-chain (approx. 32 kDa) linked by a disulfide bond analogically appears as 'H'. The B-chain, gets hooked specifically to eukaryotic cell surface facilitates toxins' internalization. The A-chain inhibits elongation factor, thus prevents 60S ribosome mediated protein synthesis, lead to cell death.

The protein synthesis inhibition involves catalytic inactivation of the ribosome by A-chain of abrin, happens through removal of an adenine from position 4 and 324 of the 28S rRNA in the 60S ribosomal subunit. The depurinated rRNA is then unable to bind protein elongation factor-2 (EF-1 and EF-2), which leads to cessation of protein synthesis, and eventual cell death. Abrin A (Sepharose nonbinding protein) and abrin C (Sepharose-binding protein) are most discerned toxalbumin. Abrin C exhibits higher toxicity in mice.

Like ricin, the ratti seeds also contain other strong hemagglutinins. Endothelial cell damage is one of the typical features of abrin toxicity. This increases capillary permeability which leads to fluid and protein leakage and consequent tissue edema *i.e.* vascular leak syndrome.

Toxicokinetics

Ingestion of jequirity beans has fatal consequences, suggests that the small amount of undigested toxin is enough to create trouble. Most of the intravenously administered abrin in mice was found in the liver, thereafter in blood, lungs, spleen, kidneys and heart. When abrin is injected *via* intraperitoneal route, it cumulates most of it abrin in liver, followed by the kidneys and blood, and abrin was commonly in unchanged form. It follows renal elimination as low molecular weight degradation products.

In the early 20th century, it had been used for homicide in many countries, including India and Sri Lanka. Needle prepared from ground seeds of *Abrus precatorius* is used to pierce in the muscular portion of the animals to kill.

Toxicity

Abrus poisoning has occurred in many animals, including dogs, poultry, wild fowl, pigs, horses, sheep, and goats. It depends upon the crushing and release of toxic principle when taken orally. Toxicity depends on route and amount of exposure.

Inhalation is the route which is most lethal followed by parenteral and oral route. Most of the human poisoning is due to ingestion of ratti seeds, either accidentally or being administered as folk medicine. Oral abrin LD_{50} in human is estimated to be 0.1–1 mg/kg body weight. The oral LD_{50} in mouse and rat is about 2.3 mg/kg body weight. On the other hand, intraperitoneal LD_{50} for abrin is 0.6 μg/kg body weight. Abrin-C is more toxic, with an LD_{50} of 0.2 μg/kg body weight in mice.

Clinical Signs and Symptoms

In human, clinical sign begin with nausea followed by abdominal pain, vomition, diarrhea, cramps, dilated pupil, fever, dehydration, anuria, sore throat, headache, hypotension, heartburn, internal bleeding of the stomach and intestines, and failure of the liver, spleen, and kidneys. The toxin damages endothelial cells, causes leakage in blood vessels, hypoalbuminemia and edema which leads to vascular system collapse, shock and death within three days or more.

Diagnosis

Due to similarities with more commonly encountered illnesses, recognition of poisoning by abrin is challenging. For its definitive confirmation, it requires epidemiological information around cases of accidental poisoning. Abrin solution loses its toxic actions when heated to temperatures of 80 °C and beyond.

The detection of ricinine and L-abrine, in urine samples of intoxicated models are suitable surrogate markers for the diagnosis of intoxication.

Inhalation of aerosolized ricin or abrin is considered the most dangerous mode of exposure. Lung lavage washing can be the most suitable clinical sample for early diagnostic testing to confirm suspected poisoning by aerosolized ricin or abrin.

Clinical Management and Prognosis

Currently, treatment for abrin poisoning is symptomatic and supportive due to lack of specific treatment protocols or antidotes.

Emesis is beneficial in animals that can vomit if instituted early after oral ingestion. Charcoal is of little significance in order to prevent its further systemic absorption. However, activated charcoal 1-4 gm/kg body weight orally and magnesium sulfate at 250 mg/kg body weight orally or 70 per cent sorbitol at 3 ml/kg body weight orally can be beneficial.

Protectants such as kaolin-pectin or sucralfate 0.25 to 2 gm three times a day orally should be used.

Adequate fluid and electrolyte therapy is of value to mitigate with hypotension. Bland diet can be of value once vomition is controlled.

Renal and liver function may not alter for initial 12 to 24 hours after oral lectin's exposure. Repeated liver and kidney function test should be adopted to let these profiles normalize. Antibiotics, lactulose (0.1 to 0.5 mg/kg body weight three times a day orally), or dietary management along with appropriate fluid therapy can be used to correct the clinical signs associated with hepatic failure. Inhalational exposure require resuscitative care *i.e.* oxygen, bronchodilators, anti-inflammatory and analgesic agents, positive-pressure ventilation along with fluid and electrolyte replacement therapy.

Abrus seeds should be kept away from the reach of children and pets. This plant is also grown for ornamental purpose; the seeds produced should not be left around. Animal feed that contain lectins should be heat-treated before they are fed. Once the symptoms are set the prognosis is guarded.

Prevention

Prior vaccination and/or prompt antitoxin antibody administration after exposure may prevent the initiation of intoxication, thus improves prognosis. Its immunotoxin has selective antitumor activity. The development of vaccine against abrin appears promising and active immunization could protect animal or human from the lethal effects of abrin poisoning. Vaccination of personnel prior to engaging in war may have its utility. More instant protection in this sense can probably be provided by antitoxins produced in sheep and horses, though they do not allow for administration in humans more than once in a lifetime. It has been noted that there is a relative paucity of research efforts to develop diagnostics and therapeutic options for abrin poisoning.

Strychnine

☆ *Nrip Kishore Pankaj and Ramesh K. Nirala*

Scientific Name

Strychnos nux vomica

Common Name

Kuchla

Strychnine is an alkaloid, isolated from the flattened seeds of *Strychnos nux vomica* and *Strychnos ignatii*. It has been used as pesticide (rodenticide, avicide, and insecticide) since few centuries. Strychnine poisoning among animals is either a result of malafide intention or accidental ingestion of baits (gopher bait) targeted for its use against rodents. The most common prey to this poisoning is dog.

Toxicokinetics

Strychnine is readily absorbed from the small intestine, distributed within 5 minutes to tissues thus can be traced less than 4 ppm at any moment in blood at any given time. It is moderately bound to plasma protein. Its half-life in human is about 10 hrs. Strychnine is readily metabolized in liver, rapidly eliminated in urine, soon after exposure. Following exposure to a sub lethal dose of strychnine, almost half of the administered dose is eliminated within 6 hours and almost complete in 48–72 hours.

Mechanism of Action

Strychnine interferes with glycine in the anterior horn of the spinal cord. Glycine is an inhibitory neurotransmitter to motor neurons and interneurons in the spinal cord. Strychnine is selective competitive antagonist which blocks the inhibitory action of glycine on its receptors in spinal cord. This initiates excessive neuronal activity thereby lead to highly agitated reflex arc. Further, mild to moderate muscle spasms followed by extreme hyperextension of limbs and body culminate in to full tetanic convulsions.

Glutamic acid is an excitatory neurotransmitter in brain that excites muscle tone, which leads to contraction. All voluntary muscles remain hyper-excitable, which gets in to vicious circle of persistent contraction at little sound or touch.

Toxicity

Strychnine is highly poisonous alkaloid for all classes of animals with oral LD_{50} 3mg/kg body weight in rat, 2mg/kg in mice, and 0.5mg/kg in cattle and dogs, 2mg/kg in cat, 5mg/kg in poultry. Presently, strychnine is used as rodenticide, avicide, and insecticide. Among animals, poisoning occurs among small animals especially in dogs either due to accidental ingestion of nontargeted bait or malicious intent out of jealousy. The onset of toxidrome can become obvious within 15 to 60 minutes following oral exposure in empty stomach, and delayed in fed animals. The toxic signs is due to increase in muscle tone due to CNS action of strychnine, thus skeletal muscles undergo simultaneous contraction.

The toxicity symptoms include restlessness, anxiety, muscle twitching and stiffness of neck. The strychnine exposed dogs' exhibit tonic convulsions with brief period of pause (relaxation), which gets progressively shorter. The animals become highly sensitive, even little stimulus like light, noise or touch during intermittent relaxation, trigger violent tonic convulsion, culminate in to hypothermia, lactic acidosis, and rhabdomyolysis. The most powerful effects are seen on the muscles of joints. Muscles involved with respiration (*i.e.* diaphragm, thoracic, and abdominal muscles) contract and eventually terminate respiration leading to death.

Strychnine exposed bird exhibit the signs of ataxia, ruffled feathers, wing droop, salivation, tremor, convulsion and death due to respiratory failure.

Postmortem Findings

Postmortem findings are usually nonspecific and exhibits marks of struggle and trauma during convulsion and suffocation associated lesions like pinpoint hemorrhages in lungs. GIT may show the presence of bait. Rigor mortis happens rapidly and persists for days. It has not been found associated to any mutagenicity, carcinogenicity, reproductive and developmental toxicity.

Diagnosis

It depends upon:

i. History of exposure to a strychnine bait in GIT

ii. Clinical signs of tetanic convulsions, seizures, hypersensitivity to external stimuli, and muscle stiffness

iii. Strychnine in the stomach content, blood, urine, or visceral organs (liver and kidney) can be quantified by gas chromatography-flame ionization detector or gas chromatography mass spectrometry.

iv. Strychnine causes rise of serum enzymes, *viz.* glutamic oxaloacetic transaminase (GOT), creatine phosphokinase (CPK), lactate dehydrogenase (LDH) as well as lactic acidosis, hyperkalemia, and leukocytosis.

v. Animal may exhibit saw horse stance similar to tetanus, thus needs to rule out.

Treatment

The treatment is more or less targeted towards restoring the vital signs symptomatically due to non availability of specific antidote. It may be approached as:

i. Barbiturates raise the threshold of spinal reflexes in animals. Thus pentobarbital is used to control strychnine-induced convulsions *i.e.* pentobarbiturate (5-15mg/kg body weight, intravenous (IV) to be repeated 4 to 8 hourly) or Diazepam (IV @0.5 to 5 mg/kg body weight in dogs; 0.5 to 1 mg/kg body weight in cats can be repeated to its effect) has muscle relaxant, anxiolytic and anticonvulsant properties.

ii. Respiration should be instituted.

iii. The muscle relaxant drugs like glyceryl guaiacolate @110mg/kg or methocarbamol @55-220mg/kg body weight, IV (ceiling dose up to 330mg/kg/day) may be used and repeated as required.

iv. Potassium permagnate or tannin may be used to lavage and neutralize strychnine in GIT following proper sedation and intubation.

v. Diuresis with 5 per cent mannitol should be opted to facilitate elimination of strychnine via urine.

vi. Ion trapping by urine acidification may be supportive to eliminate strychnine.

vii. The ambience should be kept dark, calm and warm to prevent any stimulation and hypothermia respectively.

viii. Administration of activated charcoal with sorbitol should be used to adsorb strychnine from gut.

ix. Respiration needs to be monitored for its rhythm, rate and depth along with readily available assistance to deal with severe respiratory depression.

x. Hypovolemia if any should be corrected by Ringer lactate, normal saline solution/dextrose normal saline, along with means to correct hyperthermia if any and acidosis.

Prognosis

Strychnine exposure has very rapid onset. So it is very important to deal with the poisoning to its earliest among small animals especially dogs. If we could adopt aggressive decontamination measures for first 24 hours of exposure, it has good prognosis. Any delay adversely affects and jeopardize the outcome. The prognosis for strychnine affected large animals like ruminants and horses is poor.

Cotton Seed

☆ *Nrip Kishore Pankaj and Nirbhay Kumar*

Scientific Names

Gossypium arboretum, G. herbaceum

Common Name

Cotton

"Gossypol" is yellow, crystalline, polyphenolic aldehyde. Gossypol is toxic; therefore undesirable component of the cottonseed. It is termed upon its family species gossypium and its polyphenolic chemical nature. Cottonseed is the most important source of gossypol. It is located naturally in small intercellular pigment glands in the leaves, stems, roots, and seed of cotton plants. It acts as natural pesticide as an evolved mean to protect the plant from insects and pests. The content of gossypol is high in cottonseed (6.0 per cent) followed by root bark (1.8 per cent) and leaves (0.3 per cent). The amount varies depending upon the variety and climatic conditions. During the seed processing, the ruptured glands facilitate gossypol complex with seeds' protein, thus render it non toxic. This complex formation enhances with rise in temperature. Gossypol is toxic and remains in bound and free form in seed meal. There are four species of cotton grown throughout the world.

Some Common Cotton Plants

Botanical Name	Common Name
Gossypium arboretum and *G. herbaceum*	Asian cotton
G. barbadense	Egyptian cotton
G. hirsutum	American Upland cotton

G. hirsutum is grown predominantly by occupying over 90 per cent world share. India is 2nd producer of cotton after China.

Cotton seed is source of protein and oil. It contains 23 per cent of high quality protein and about 20 per cent oil, which includes both the saturated and unsaturated fatty acids, therefore healthy for heart. But its utility is restricted due to the presence of gossypol. Cottonseed hull (hard outer shell) is quality palatable roughage for ruminant. The nutritive value of cottonseed hull is comparable to quality grass hay. It is also a valuable digestive aid. After dehulling, the available seed meal is rich source (40 per cent) of quality protein containing all the amino acids in good proportions. Cottonseed oil is rich in tocopherol which inhibits rancidity and thus contributes to its longer shelf life. Apart from protein and oil, cottonseed meal is also rich in minerals, especially higher in phosphorous.

Gossypol is used traditionally in Mexico for scalp infection, dysentery, gonorrhea and as antiseptic. It is known to possess antiviral, antipsoriasis, antikeratitic and neoplastic activity. It is also used as appetite suppressant and anti-microbial agent. Gossypol has been used as male contraceptive in China since long with the claim that it does not affect men's hormonal balance. However there is some claim that prolonged use of gossypol may lead to impotency. Recently, gossypol has been claimed to possess anticancer activity against prostate cancer, breast cancer cells both *in vitro* and *in vivo* as well as metastatic adrenal cancer.

Low concentrations of gossypol and other cotton toxins from cottonseed have been reported to improve the effectiveness of insecticidal agents against domestic insects including cockroaches, termites and ants *i.e.* the insecticidal agents which are ineffective in control of social insects alone are reported to be effective when used in conjunction with the cotton toxins. Gossypol can be reduced at moist pressure cooking during 60 minutes cooking period at 15 psi, and 250° F.

Toxicity

Gossypol can enter in to cells and inhibits many dehydrogenase enzymes including protein kinase C. It is soluble in acetone, chloroform, ether, ethanol, isopropanol and methyl ethyl ketone (butanone). It is partly soluble in crude vegetable oils and insoluble in water and hexane. Gossypol primarily affects heart, liver, reproductive tract and kidney in monogastric animals such as pigs. Gossypol toxicity leads to kidney malfunction depicted by hypokalemia which leads to symptoms of fatigue, muscle weakness and ultimately paralysis. The toxicity of gossypol can be reversed if discontinued and properly supplemented with potassium. Among cattle and sheep, free ingested gossypol gets complexed with protein in rumen therefore can tolerate its higher levels.

Young calves and lambs are susceptible to gossypol toxicity similar to monogastric animals as their rumen is not fully functional and therefore fail to bind free gossypol. Increased intake of feed containing cotton seed meal by milch cows could compromise the protective function of rumen in preventing gossypol toxicity. Swine, guinea pigs and rabbits are most sensitive to gossypol toxicity. Cats and dogs have intermediate sensitivity to gossypol followed by poultry, mice and rats.

Clinical Signs and Symptoms

Two types of clinical syndromes have been observed, especially in young animals.

1. The syndrome resemble heart attack in calves and lambs. These animals are apparently healthy with good appetite and among best in group, but succumb. Such calves fail to survive the stressful situation *i.e.* transit.
2. The other syndrome resembles pneumonia characterized by chronic laboured breathing. Here again heart is affected, the lungs gets engorged with fluid and thus render breathing tough. These animals do not respond to antibiotics. Animal is depressed, off fed and may die gradually.

The common symptoms of toxicity includes weakness, depression, loss of appetite, difficult breathing, blood in urine, inflammation of intestines and reproductive problem. The permissible limits of gossypol in animal and human feed are as mentioned in table below:

Permissible Limits of Gossypol Feed

Animals	*Maximum Gossypol Allowed in Feed*
Swine	100 ppm
Calves and Lambs (less than 4 months)	100ppm
Adult cattle	800ppm
Human food	450ppm

Clinical Pathology

Increased erythrocyte fragility thus decreased packed cell volume. Liver enzymes are also elevated.

Lesions

In the case of sudden death, may not show any lesions. Although, gross lesions due chronic heart failure includes:

- ☆ Fluid in the thoracic and peritoneal cavities are uniformly heavy and wet.
- ☆ Edema of the lymph nodes, mesentery, intestine, and other organs.
- ☆ The pericardial sac contains clear to red-tinged fluid with fibrin clots.
- ☆ Heart is enlarged and flabby with dilated ventricles and edematous valves.
- ☆ Streaked, pale, or mottled cardiac musculature.
- ☆ Liver may be pale, swollen and friable
- ☆ Kidneys are congested and spleen is pale

Histopathology

- ☆ Myocardial degeneration
- ☆ Centrilobular hepatic necrosis and congestion,
- ☆ Pulmonary edema.
- ☆ Renal tubular necrosis, abomasitis, and enteritis have also been seen.

Treatment

As such antidote is not available, it is better to avoid any such feed to animal except the limits mentioned in table. It take several weeks to months for an exposed animal back to normal, if animals are not severely affected can be managed in stress free situation.

Nitrate and Nitrite

☆ *Nrip Kishore Pankaj and Shahid Prawez*

Nitrogen is vital for a life to exist, which is provided by plants in the form of nitrate and nitrite. Nitrate poisoning among livestock happens when they consume too much of high nitrate containing green forage and the animal system fails to reduce nitrate into amino acids and protein. Poisoning can also happen when animals eat too much urea or nitrogen fertilizer spilled in the field or left where the animals can find it. These fertilizers are palatable, especially to cattle. Nitrate or nitrite is the integral part of all plants; its excessive accumulation does occur in fodder plants which grow under any kind of stress even in the cases of excessive fertilizers application. The fertilizers usually contain nitrogen in the form of ammonia and urea, which is converted in to its nitrate form by the soil microbes. As nitrate form of nitrogen is highly soluble, easily absorbed by plants, reduced to ammonium form and assimilated in to amino acids and proteins. The whole episode is called nitrate reduction. This happens in the roots (bermuda grass), leaves and stem of plants (sorghum).

Potential Nitrate Accumulator Weeds and Forage Plants

Botanical Name	Common Names	Botanical Name	Common Names
Avena sativa	Oat, jai	*Triticum aestivum*	Wheat
Zea mays	Maize	*Brassica* spp.	Rape, Turnip
Glycine max	Soyabean	*Beta vulgaris*	Beet
Hordeum spp.	Barley	*Linum usitatissimum*	Flax
Pennisetum typhoides	Pearl millet	*Secale cereale*	Rye
Medicago sativa	Alfalfa, lucerne	*Sorghum vulgare* (spp.)	Jwar
Melilotus officinalis	Sweetclover	*Silybum marianum*	Milk thistle
Amaranthus spp.	Pigweed	*Solanum* spp.	Nightshades
Chenopodium spp.	Lambsquarters	*Rumex* spp.	Docks
Helianthus annuus	Annual sunflower		

Sources of Toxicity

i. Along with the factors mentioned above, the livestock may consume nitrate fertilizers, leading to accidental toxicity among ruminants.

ii. The decaying organic matter from crop field may trickle in the well around, may contain as high as 1700-3000 ppm, is an important source of poisoning.

iii. Animal wastes from butcher drain also raise nitrate level in water to toxic level.

iv. Regular use of nitrite, organic nitrates in therapy may also be hazardous.

Factor affecting Toxicity

A. Environmental Factors

i. The stalks of the plant contain higher nitrate concentration with respect to other parts of plants, although depends primarily on the nitrate concentration in soil. Younger plants usually contain greater nitrate concentration.

ii. Drought stress: High temperatures or low humidity, cold temperatures, hail damage and frost may slow or stop plant growth and cause nitrates to accumulate. When the fodder crop is exposed to enough moisture and higher environmental temperature, undergoes photorespiration, this suppresses assimilation of carbon into carbohydrates, rather produce CO_2. This facilitates nitrate accumulation in plants. On the other hand when enough nitrogen remains present along with deficiency of moisture in the soil, plants take up nitrates in relatively concentrated form. The build up of nitrates in soil also happen due to excessive application of poultry litter or animal manure. Plants need water to get it utilized but fail due to lack of enough water, thus facilitate accumulation of nitrates. After a heavy rainfall, plant growth lets nitrate accumulation reduce in plants therefore harvest should be delayed for 3 to 4 days after the rain.

iii. Suppressed photosynthesis especially in cloudy days and highly dense plant populations may also facilitate to accumulate higher nitrates content in plants.

iv. Application of herbicide suppresses the conversion and assimilation of nitrates thereby responsible for accumulation of nitrate in plants.

v. Photosynthesis may be suppressed in tissues that could cause nitrates to accumulate in plants by interfering with nitrate reduction, protein synthesis or the manufacture and translocation of carbohydrates.

vi. Micro and macro minerals *i.e.* molybdenum, copper, iron, magnesium, sulfur or manganese are involved in the enzyme system of plants for reducing nitrates in to amino acid and proteins. This may cause nitrates to accumulate in plants.

B. Animal Factors

The toxicity due to nitrate/nitrite depends upon various factors *viz.*

i. Among cattle the ruminal microflora convert nitrate to nitrite at rapid rate and later in to ammonia which is less efficient and rate limiting. This facilitates absorption of nitrite ion in to blood circulation and responsible for methemoglobinemia.

ii. Sheep has better conversion of nitrite in to ammonia, therefore less vulnerable to its toxicity. The sheep are less sensitive to nitrate in ration due to their slower intake rate and shorter elimination half-life (4.2 hr as compared to 9 hr in cattle).

iii. Nitrate toxicosis in horses and pigs is rare owing to absence of nitrate conversion in to nitrite. However, highly susceptible to direct oral nitrite toxicity as they lack the mechanism to convert nitrite in to ammonia.

iv. Hungry animals are more vigorous in consuming forage (toxic feed) and ruminal microbes fail to quickly adapt in converting the nitrite to ammonia leads to serious toxicosis.

v. Ruminants consuming fodders with high carbohydrate (grains) tolerate better to higher nitrate and nitrite levels with respect to those that are not. This is due to carbohydrate mediated energy, which facilitates ruminal organism, convert nitrite to ammonia.

Poisoning

Nitrate is one of the most oxidised forms of nitrogen in nature. It is non-volatile and remains in non-ensiled plants after harvesting, curing and baling. It is safe to feed forage containing 0.5-1 per cent nitrate (on a dry-matter basis) to healthy ruminants. In healthy cattle, the nitrate consumed in normal forages is converted to nitrite then in to ammonia followed by amino acids and finally proteins. In the case of forage, toxicity generally occurs when apparently healthy cattle consume forage containing 1.76 per cent or more nitrate ion on a dry matter basis.

Nitrite ion is ten times more reactive as compared to nitrate. Although nitrate acts as source of nitrite, which is responsible for met-hemoglobinemia and respiratory toxidrome.

Nitrates play important role in inducing vasodilatation in addition to met-hemoglobinemia which compromise oxygen carrying capacity of haemoglobin, lead to peripheral circulatory collapse. This may be a cause of abortion along with some signs of nitrate toxicity in herd such as bluish unpigmented areas of the skin or mucous membranes and death. When met-hemoglobinemia reaches 30 to 40 per cent level, symptoms of nitrate poisoning appear. The most common symptom of nitrate intoxication include dyspnoea, rapid rate of breathing, bluish membrane, muscular tremor, weakness, exercise intolerance, in coordination, diarrhoea, frequent urination, chocolate coloured blood and collapse. Death supervenes when methemoglobinemia reaches 80 to 90 per cent. Death may ensue within 30 to 240 minutes following appearance of symptoms.

The acute LD_{50} of Sodium Nitrate and Nitrite for cattle is 650-750mg/kg and 150-170 mg/kg body weight respectively.

Presence of excess ammonia in the rumen may happen in nitrate poisoning. This may forms a complex chemical salt at pH 6.2-6.4 in presence of magnesium and phosphorus. This prevents its absorption and cause grass tetany.

Mechanism of Toxicity

Soon after entry in rumen, over 25 per cent of nitrate is converted to nitrite by microbial reductase in anaerobic ambience. This requires copper, iron and magnesium @ pH 5.6-5.8. Nitrite is further converted in to hydroxylamine (in presence of copper, iron and magnesium) and finally ammonia (in presence of magnesium and manganese). Nitrite reductase is inhibited by nitrate. Nitrite accumulation in the rumen occurs when nitrate ingestion and reduction to nitrite exceeds that of nitrite reduction to ammonia due to difference in the level of reductive enzyme. As such some fraction of nitrite formed in the rumen enters the blood circulation where it oxidizes hemoglobin (ferrous Fe^{+2} ion) to methemoglobin (ferric Fe^{+3} ion). Usually, when nitrite level raises in blood the ferric iron in methemoglobin is converted back to functional ferrous iron in haemoglobin by NADPH-dependent reduction. When NADPH-dependent reduction gets overwhelmed, causes methemoglobinemia (Figure 9.1). This destroys the oxygen-carrying capacity of affected haemoglobin (met-hemoglobinemia). Mild symptom of poisoning *i.e.* exercise intolerance may appear when methemoglobin levels reach 30 per cent to 40 per cent, whereas methemoglobinemia @ 80 per cent or over are fatal.

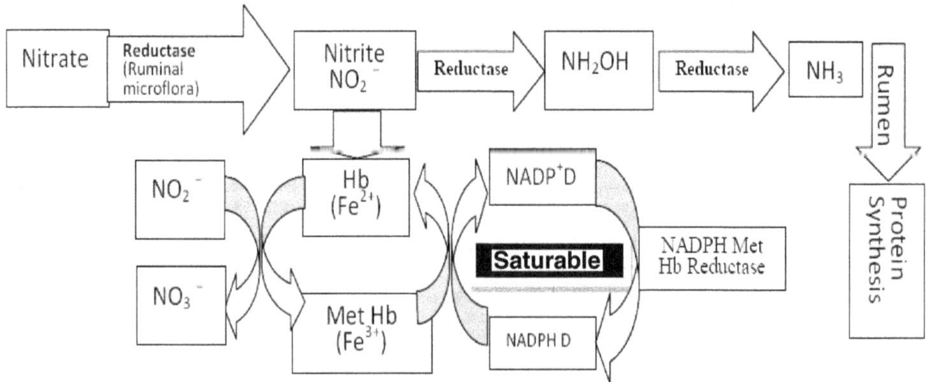

Figure 9.1: Normal Pathway of Nitrate in Ruminants.

When the nitrite reductase reaction is over whelmed, it starts of NO_2^- pouring in blood circulation, leading to methemoglobinemia (MetHb). When conversion of MetHb to Hb gets saturated due to insufficient NADPH-MetHb reductase, results into respiratory toxidrome.

Nitrate and nitrite are vasoactive compounds as well. It induces nitric oxide synthesis in the endothelium of blood vessel, which facilitate dephosphorylation of GTP *via* Guanyl cyclase. Consequently myosin light chain kinase (**MLCK**) is also dephosphorylated and thus gets relaxed. This reduces vascular tone, further compromises delivery of oxygen to the tissues *i.e.* hypotension (Figure 9.2).

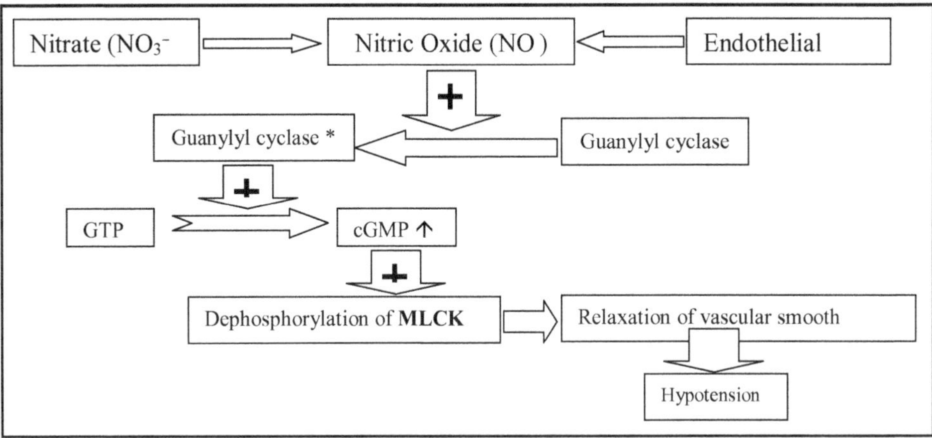

Figure 9.2: Smooth Muscles Relaxation of Blood Vessels in Nitrate/Nitrite Toxicity by NO Genesis.

When nitrate is consumed accidently in large amount by the animals, it acts somewhat similar to salt toxicity. It is manifested by altered osmotic situation and irritation in GIT mucosa, kidney and urinary tract.

Clinical Signs and Symptoms

Initial symptoms are marked by irritation of GIT *i.e.* salivation, diarrhoea and abdominal pain. Later phase of symptoms are characterized by dyspnoea in acute cases. It gets progressively severe to marked respiratory distress, open mouth breathing, followed by violent respiratory movement along with extreme apprehension. A rapid and weak heart beat (over 150/min), hypothermia, muscular weakness, staggering gait, muscular tremors, cyanosis of mucous membranes followed by marked dilation of pupils appears commonly in chronology. Chocolate colour of the blood is characteristic of nitrate poisoning. Death may ensue within 3 to 4 hours of the onset of dyspnoea.

In subacute or chronic nitrate poisoning, abortion is usually accompanied or preceded by some evidence of nitrate poisoning in the animals, including cyanosis of albino areas of the skin or mucous membranes. Reproductive problems may be prevented if nitrate-containing feeds are gradually introduced into the diet and the nitrate level in the total ration dry matter is maintained below 1.76 per cent. In chronic cases, dyspnoea, anorexia, poor weight gain and reduction in milk production is commonly observed.

Post-mortem Findings

There is severe hyperaemia and stripping of the stomach and intestinal linings corresponding to hemorrhagic gastroenteritis, pinpointed haemorrhages and accumulation of blood in the stomach wall. Blood become dark red or chocolate brown that clots poorly along with brownish cast to all tissues is typical of nitrate poisoning; however there is no pathognomic lesion in nitrate/nitrite toxicity.

Diagnosis

Diagnosis is based upon observed clinical signs, possible exposure to toxic plants and feeds or water, post-mortem and laboratory findings. A quick test for detection of nitrate toxicity in fodder is the diphenylamine spot test. It contains diphenylamine salt (0.1 gram) dissolved in sulfuric acid (30 ml-36N). One single drop of this reagent is placed on a freshly split plant stem. Appearance of dark blue colour within 5 seconds is confirmatory to presence of nitrate in the sample. Any delay in colour development is indicative of nontoxic level of nitrate. Nitrate stays longer in aqueous humor in the cases of toxicity, which is of diagnostic value as well if found over 20ppm.

There are few toxicants which interfere with oxygen carrying capacity of blood *i.e.* carbon monoxide, carbon dioxide, warfarin, cyanide, chlorates, hypotensives *etc.* needs to be differentially diagnosed.

Treatment

Suspected material should be removed immediately from heard. The animals should be handled properly to avoid stress mediated aggravation, dyspnoea and death of the intoxicated animals.

i. Methylene blue is the specific antidote administered IV @ 5 to 15 mg/kg BW as 1 per cent (up to 22 mg/kg body weight) solution in NSS. Depending upon improvement lower doses can be repeated 6-8 hourly.

   Ruminant can tolerate higher dose, although overdosing may lead to methemoglobinemia further. Methylene blue acts as an electron carrier for an NADPII-dependent system thus reduce methemoglobin to oxygen carrying haemoglobin (Figure 9.3).

   Methylene blue is most effective in ruminants and human. Tissues in the methylene blue treated animals become stained and the urine becomes dark green. Therefore treated animals should not be sold for slaughter for 6 months. Other dyes such as tolonium blue are effective for the purpose but have a narrow therapeutic index

ii. Hay or some other low nitrate forage should be fed to dilute the nitrate and/or nitrite in the rumen. Rumen lavage with cold water and oral penicillin may suppress the continuous reduction of nitrate to nitrite.

iii. Ascorbic acid being a reducing agent @5-20 mg/kg body weight may be used for the purpose *via* intravenous route.

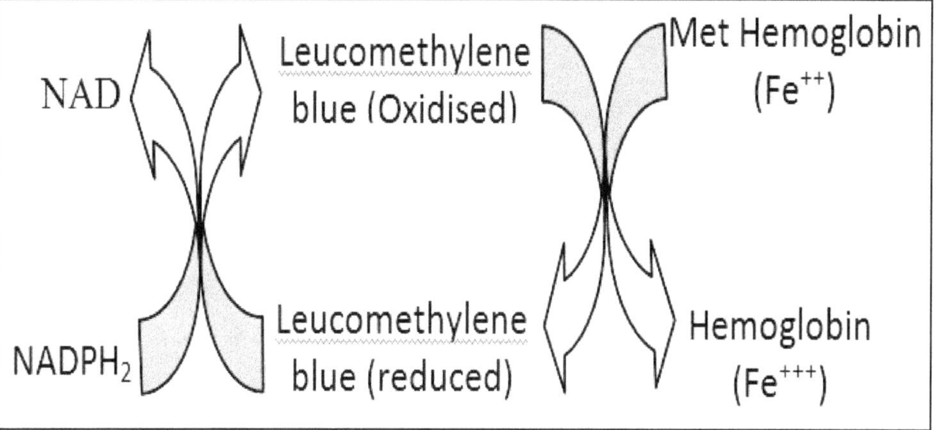

Figure 9.3: Mechanism of Regeneration of Haemoglobin Aided by Methylene Blue (Schematic Diagram).

iv. Blood transfusion along with oxygen therapy.

v. Shock therapy in hypotension.

vi. Enough water supply to dilute the toxicant.

vii. Saline purgative and mineral oil.

viii. Vitamin and trace minerals along with iodine may be helpful.

ix. Administration of α adrenergic agonist (oxygen demand) or antagonist (complicate hypotension) should be avoided.

Preventive Measure

i. Feeding hungry animals on dry hay or mature grass and well-dried cereal hays before letting free access to immature cereal crops or root-crop tops.

ii. Preventing hungry animals from grazing recently sprayed weeds and highly fertilised forages.

iii. Not letting graze high-nitrate pastures or crops for 7 days after periods of rainfall, cloudy days, frosts, or high temperatures that cause wilting.

iv. Feeding risky fodder in small amounts diluted with safe feed, preferably high-carbohydrate feed such as grain, gradually increasing the amount fed to ruminants.

v. Ensuring that water does not contain high levels of nitrates;

vi. Another option for reducing the risk of nitrate/nitrite poisoning is to harvest and feed high-nitrate forages as silage. This is because nitrate levels are reduced by the fermentation process when feed is ensiled.

Ipomoea

☆ *Nrip Kishore Pankaj and Pawan K. Verma*

Scientific Names

Ipomoea carnea, I. purge, I. orizabensis, I. violacea

Common Names

Besharam, Thethar, Pink Morning Glory

Pink Morning Glory or *Ipomoea* belongs to family Convolvulaceae and is distributed widely all over the world including India. It has over 500 species including *Ipomoea carnea, I. purge, I. orizabensis, I. violacea.* The shrub of *I. carnea* is perennial and up to 2.5 m tall, of which, branches are ascending and contain milky juice. The stem of *I.carnea* is erect, woody, hairy, greenish and cylindrical in shape, monopodially branched, and bears alternate leaves. Some of its species are climbers. These plants has beautiful trumpet shaped white to purple flowers. It can grow in marshy area, and withstand the drought easily, and remains green. *I. carnea* is a weed in pastures; animals usually don't favour it, but are compelled during fodder scarcity. Some animal may even develop taste for it as well. Its seed are toxic and it can be hazardous to cattle.

Ipomoea carnea plants do possess some medicinal value as well. It is claimed to be used in leucoderma, as aphrodisiac, purgative and cathartic. It contains marsilin like constituent which has sedative and anticonvulsant properties. An anticarcinogenic and oxytoxic glycosidic saponin has also been purified from *I. carnea.*

Toxicity

The toxic principle in Ipomoea is strongly irritant resin *i.e.* Jalapin/Scammonin in *Ipomoea orizabensis,* turpethin in *I. turpethum,* pharbitisin in *I. hederaeceae,* that produce catharsis in acute cases. Some species of *Ipomoea* also contain hallucinogenic compounds like lysergic acid and indole alkaloids. The toxicity of *I.carnea* is more common in small ruminants such as goats and sheeps. In sub acute cases in goats, the signs of *I.carnea* intoxication are mostly of nervous origin; which include depression, staggering gait, muscle tremors, ataxia, nervousness and weight loss.

Wistar rats subjected to Ipomoea exposure leads to leukocytosis, anemia, elevated serum Aspartate Amino Transferase activity and decrease in albumin level. The toxins in *I.carnea* are the indolizidine alkaloid swainsonine and the nortropane alkaloids calystegines. The dihydroxynortropane alkaloids are thought to be responsible for these toxic effects of *I.carnea,* potentiated by calystegines.

Lysosomal Storage Disease (LSD)

Swainsonine, but not calystegines, are produced by fungi that live epiphytically with *I.carnea*. Swainsonine is a powerful neurotoxic indolizidine alkaloid, inhibits lysosomal α-mannosidase and Golgi mannosidase II, causing excessive carbohydrate accumulation within lysosomes known as lysosomal storage disease. This leads to lysosomal accumulation of incompletely processed oligosaccharides, vacuolation and cellular death. In goats, such damage is especially severe in the CNS. This vacuolar degeneration can be seen in other organs such as thyroid, liver, pancreas, and kidneys. *Ipomoea carnea* is one of the plants capable of accumulating swainsonine, along with plants of the genera Astragalus, Oxytropis, Sida, and Swainsona. Regular consumption of *I.carnea* causes generalized weakness, loss of body weight, alopecia, locomotor disturbance, loss of reflexes, intero-hepato-nephropathy, muscle tremors, ataxia, posterior paresis, paralysis and even death. Neurological signs, characteristic of cerebellar and brainstem alterations such as hypermetria, ataxia, and intention tremors are common in exposed animals along with severe weight loss. It may cause adverse effects in cattle, horses and goats including neurological alterations including failure to take and swallow feed. Commonly LSDs are genetic disorders; however it can be induced due to consumption of toxic plants like Locoweeds *i.e. Astragalus, Oxytropis* spp. and *I. carnea* in goats.

Affected animals exhibit ataxia with head tremors and nystagmus. Calystegines inhibit lysosomal α-galactosidase and β-glycosidase and these alkaloids potentiate the lesions produced by swansonine, however, it is unknown how the nortropane alkaloids contribute to the toxicity of *I. carnea*, particularly in a ruminant model.

Swainsonine's mediated inhibition of Golgi mannosidase II, leads to changes in the synthesis, processing, and transport of glycoproteins, which causes dysfunction in hormones and membrane receptors and leads to alterations in endocrine and reproductive functions.

Teratological Effects

The pregnant rats subjected to prenatal oral exposure of *I.carnea*, develop organ-specific toxicity of thyroid, pancreas, liver and kidneys among off springs, characterized by cytoplasmic vacuolization. Further, it leads to spleenomegaly and atrophy of thymus in pups and decline in body weight. Feeding of aqueous extract of *I.carnea* leads to decline in 3,4-dihydroxyphenylacetic acid and increase in vanilmandelic acid levels in striatum, cortex and hypothalamus in a diffusive manner. This indicated decline in dopamine and enhanced norepinephrine activity in pups. Administration of 7.5 g/kg body weight of *I.carnea* leaves to pregnant goats, resulted in fetal death, abortion, stillbirths, cytoplasmic vacuolation in the fetal CNS, and structural and functional changes in the offspring.

Clinical Signs and Symptoms

The severity of toxicosis depends upon the amount of the plants leaves or else consumed. *Ipomoea* consumption at lower doses usually leads to diarrhea, which may get aggravated to drastic purgation at higher doses. Other symptoms include nausea, salivation, mydriasis, ataxia, staggering gait followed by hallucination, delayed reflexes, prostration, paralysis of limbs, hypotension and death. In sub acute poisoning, sheep and goats exposed to Ipomoea leaves exhibit clinical signs like depression, staggering gait, muscle tremors, ataxia, nervousness, and weight loss. Dams that ingest *I. carnea* during gestation are less concerned to newborns after birth. It can compromise kid's ability to learn and retain spatial memory. Kids exposed *in utero* to *I. carnea* are low in vigor at birth, suffer of late development, if the kid survived. Kids from *Ipomoea* exposed dams had difficulty in standing, suckling, and in recognizing their mother hours after birth.

Post-mortem Findings

Apparently, there is no specific lesion due to Ipomoea poisoning in any organ, however histopathological examination exhibits vacuolar degeneration in liver, thyroid, kidney and pancreas. Lung becomes oedematous along with haemorrhage in heart.

Diagnosis and Treatment

Diagnosis more or less depends upon the history of consumption of this plant or presence of plant materials in gastrointestinal tract. The treatment for *Ipomoea* poisoning is nonspecific. General line of detoxification therapy should be followed along with supportive care and management. Rumenotomy may be required to remove the plant material from absorption further. Saline purgation or gastric lavage may be opted along with proper rehydration therapy.

Kaner

☆ *Nrip Kishore Pankaj and Rajinder Raina*

Scientific Name

Nerium oleander

Common Name

Kaner

Kaner (*Nerium oleander*) is an ornamental evergreen densely branched and commonly grown garden plant. It has leathery, pointed, long and narrow leaves along with pink to white flowers in bunches. It belongs to family Apocyanaceae, which also includes *Nerium indicum*, *Thevetia peruviana*, and *Apocynum spp*. These plants contain glycosides which produce cardiac toxicity. There are some other plant which are important source of cardiac glycosides, includes *Digitalis spp* (foxglove), *Convallaria majalis, Asclepias spp*. and *Kalanchoe spp*. The dried or fresh leaves of *Nerium* are highly toxic to animals due to its glycosidic toxins. It is cardiac glycoside, when consumed, causes serious gastroenteritis and sudden death due to cardiac failure. All parts of Oleander (twig, pod and leaves) are highly toxic and hazardous owing to chances of exposure to the livestock especially due to immaturity and accidental ingestion. The cardiac glycosides containing plants are commonly bitter therefore, animals usually avoid such vegetations. However, the plants' clipping mixed with fodder, intentionally or unintentionally usually results in to its exposure and toxicity. The animals may get exposed to its toxicity due to consumption of pond water wherein plants' clippings are disposed. Dogs are also susceptible to oleander toxicity.

Toxicity

Oleandrin and neriin are two of the major highly toxic cardiac glycosides are found in all parts of the kaner plant. These two of the toxicant are similar to the toxin found in Foxglove plant (*Digitalis spp*). These toxins have similar action *i.e.* positive inotropy and negative chronotropy. Most symptoms from oleander poisoning are cardiac and gastrointestinal in nature and appear four hours after the ingestion. The signs of toxicity may take 8 to 24 hours to become evident following exposure. Oleandrin has been found in milk of cow. It is assumed to be cleared from milk after five days of last exposure.

Oleander is one of the most toxic plants. Dry leaves of oleander can be lethal to large animals like horse and cattle at the dose of 0.005 per cent of the body weight. It can be lethal at the dose of 0.015 per cent of body weight in sheep that amounts to be 2-3 leaves. One leaf can be lethal to normal adult human. The gravity of toxicity of oleander can be observed in table below.

Animal	LD_{50} *(mg/kg bwt)*	Number of Dry Oleander Leaves
Horse	26	7-8
Cattle	45	11-12

Mechanism of Toxic Action

The cardiac glycosides oleandrin and neriin, inhibit this plasmalemmal Na^+/K^+ATPase, which is similar to digitalis glycosides. The plasmalemmal Na^+/K^+ ATPase pump is essential to maintain electrolyte balance in cardiac cells and therefore vital for cardiac function. This results in to accumulation of sodium within and potassium outside the cardiac cell. This initiates the cascade of calcium release, positive ionotrophy, thus heart block by interfering vagal tone.

Animals with digitalis like toxicosis have electrocardiographic abnormalities of sluggish AV conduction, followed by missed beats, later progressive change in ST segment results in to escape beats and ventricular arrhythmias. Oleander toxins are also directly toxic and affect the sympathetic system, leading directly to the tachyarrhythmia. This leads to an increase in PR interval, decreased QRS-T span and T wave flattening or inversion. These abnormalities are reflected as ventricular dysrhythmias, tachyarrhythmias, bradycardia, and heart block. These clinical manifestations are the result of both increased vagotonia and direct cardiac glycoside toxicity.

Animals exposed to oleander, exhibit convulsion (central) and tremor (peripheral nervous system). Livestock exposed to oleander may have diarrhea and can have large amounts of fluid in the bowel. Gastroenteritis is more common in the toxicity of kaner as compared to digoxin in human. The common poisoning symptoms due to the toxicity of kaner exposure included nausea, vomition, cramping, bloody diarrhea, burning sensation around mouth, salivation, drowsiness, dizziness, confusion, weakness, visual disturbance and mydriasis. Most symptoms from oleander poisoning are directed-to cardiac and gastrointestinal system.

Clinical Signs and Symptoms

Oleander is extremely toxic plant which affects heart and gastrointestinal tract in all types of animals following exposure. Owing to severe cardiac effects, the animals (cattle and horses) may be found dead in per-acute cases of exposure. The gravity of toxicity depends upon the dose and usually exhibits the symptoms within 2 to 8 hours of exposure leading to colic, weakness, ruminal atony, profuse salivation and vomiting in some species. It may start with bradycardia initially, followed by tachycardia and ventricular arrhythmia. Affected animal may remain lethargic and uncomfortable. The exposed animals later show pupilary dilation, tremors, hyper urination, cyanosis, excitement, intermittent convulsions, depression, dyspnea and coma before death within 2 to 48 hours following the onset of signs. Hyperkalemia is common toxic syndrome, linked to heart cell damage.

Postmortem Lesions

The lesion may not be found among animals exposed to oleander in peracute cases. In some cases bowel may be filled up with fluid along with congestion and necrosis in heart muscles. Horses may exhibit lesions associated with mild form of pulmonary edema. Pericardium and body cavity may be filled with fluid along with multifocal myocardial degeneration and necrosis.

Diagnosis

It depends initially upon circumstantial evidence and history of exposure which may be facilitated by presence of the plant materials in the ingesta and or around the premises. Oleander glycosides give cross reaction between the different types of cardiac glycosides. Thin layer chromatography (TLC) and high-performance liquid chromatography (HPLC) with mass spectroscopy can be used for confirmatory diagnosis for the presence of these glycosides in various body fluid and ingesta.

Treatment

The attempt should be directed to avoid further exposure to the toxicity. Initial approach is to evacuate the stomach after exposure to kaner and induce emesis depending upon suitability at an earliest, thereafter or else adsorbent should be considered.

- ☆ Activated charcoal or a resin *i.e.* cholestyramine may be repeatedly utilized. This also takes care of breaking the chain of enterohepatic recycling of oleander toxin.

- ☆ The treatment of oleander poisoning is commonly targeted as in the toxicity of digitalis and aimed to stabilize the subject hemodynamically. The balance of electrolyte should be observed carefully; especially potassium supplementation must be avoided in hyperkalemic cases.

- ☆ Any solution containing calcium may further aggravate the cardiac disturbance therefore contraindicated.

- ☆ The use of anticholinergic drug like atropine is usually restricted to toxicity induced bradycardia in initial 24 hours of exposure. Atropine therapy in horse may result in to gut impaction therefore needs to be administered *via* slow drip (IV). The intention is to regulate the effect of atropine only up to correction in heart rate, and or sluggishness of gut to avoid paralytic gut stasis.

☆ Later, if the animal survives first 24 hours, suffers from tachyarrythmia due to predominant sympathetic (nervous) system activation. Propranolol, phenytoin, procainamide and lidocaine may be useful in these cases.

☆ Flunixin may be useful to horses suffering from colic and diarrhea due to kaner exposure.

Datura

☆ *Nrip Kishore Pankaj and Ramesh K. Nirala*

Scientific Name

Datura spp.

Common Names

Jimson weed, Angel's trumpet

Datura spp is commonly cultivated for its flower and fruit used in certain rituals in India. It is also found as weed in gardens, crop fields and dry area close to livestock confinement and commonly linked to malicious poisoning among animals and humans in India. Few genera of the family *Solanaceae* such as *Datura stramonium, Datura metel, D. tatula, D fastuosa, D, alba, D. metel, Atropa belladonna, Hyoscyamus niger, Solanum nigrum etc.* are toxic owing to the presence of tropane group of alkaloids. All of these plants are potentially toxic and may cause sporadic poisoning among animals, however, plant belonging to genus Datura appears to be more hazardous to animals.

Toxic Principles

The toxic principles included alkaloid like daturine (a mixture of atropine and hyoscamine), scopolamine (hyoscine) and solanine which have strong anticholinergic properties, particularly concentrated in the seeds as compared to all other parts of the plant. The toxic level of tropane alkaloids is 0.15 mg/kg body weight. Cattle may be killed from ingestion of plants at 0.06 per cent to 0.09 per cent of body weight.

Mechanism of Action

Tropane alkaloids are muscarinic receptor antagonists; compete with acetylcholine (ACh) for the binding site on the muscarinic receptors. This prevents the Ach binding at muscarinic receptors in body system *viz.* all smooth and cardiac muscle, gland cells, in peripheral ganglia and in the CNS. High dose of atropine may block nicotinic receptor sites at autonomic ganglia and neuromuscular junction.

Toxicity

Rabbits, rats, guinea pigs and poultry possess atropine-hydrolases, which help them inactivate the tropane alkaloids, thus they are relatively resistant to tropane alkaloids. Horses and pigs are most sensitive to tropane alkaloids.

The course of disease may be as short as minutes or hours and is usually less than 1.5 days. In cases of acute poisoning, common clinical signs following ingestion of the datura seed include tachycardia, dilatation of pupil, photophobia, dry mouth, dysphagia, dry and hot skin, incoordination, disorientation, convulsions, delirium and coma in human. In animals these symptoms are rare. Altered salivation and ruminal atony among cattle can be noticed. For horses, the predominant sign of intoxication is severe and intractable impaction or colic. Equines exposed to Datura seed intoxication lead to symptoms like anorexia, hyper excitability, staggers, muscular spasms, frequent urination and mydriasis impaired vision progressing to convulsive seizures, rigor and coma preceding death. Under some conditions this can result in epidemic incidences of colic.

The post mortem lesions are scarce and non specific however, congestion of oesophagus, stomach, duodenum and other organs may be found. The plant materials may be found in gastrointestinal tract. Haemorrhage in brain, stomach and intestine may be observed.

Treatment

Datura has anticholinergic properties; it induces generalized atony in gastrointestinal tract, leads to colic in equines. It should be treated as per symptoms, which includes water by nasogastric tube, laxative ($MgSO_4$), cisapride per os, polyionic fluid by IV infusion at the rate of 4 ml/kg/h, and analgesic such as flunixin. This therapy should be followed until sign of discomfort is resolved.

Atropine is commonly used in veterinary practice for the treatment of organophosphorus and carbamates poisoning. This practice may demand extra care owing to the probability of colic in the horses. It is also used for the remedy of chronic obstructive pulmonary disease in horses. It has been found that the horses are especially sensitive to gastrointestinal atony on administration of atropine.

The use of specific antagonists to reverse muscarinic blockade is of vital importance among horses. This can be mitigated by using reversible acetylcholine esterase inhibiters like neostigmine and physostigmine. Although, Neostigmine (is a quarternary compound, remains ionized) is commonly used drug in veterinary medicine, it doesn't cross through blood brain barrier. Eserine (phytostigmine) is a tertiary compound (alkaloid), remains relatively non ionized, readily crosses through blood brain barrier, therefore better choice to treat tropane alkaloids poisoning in human. Swift antidotal action of Eserine abolishes symptoms such as delirium and coma in human. The same treatment may be considered for horses as well. Eserine is rapidly metabolized; therefore require frequent (1–2 hourly) dosing. Eserine is a potent drug having narrow therapeutic index. Of the natural cholinomimetic alkaloids, only arecoline and pilocarpine are not ionized.

Chapter 10

Oxalate Containing Plants

☆ *Kasturi Devi, Vijeyta Tiwari and Swatantra K. Singh*

Oxalic acid is one of the common anti-nutrients found in plants. Oxalic acid is an organic dicarboxylic acid that occurs in two forms: soluble and insoluble oxalates. Soluble oxalate usually forms with monovalent counter ions such as sodium (Na+), potassium (K^+) and ammonium (NH^{4+}), whereas insoluble oxalate forms with divalent calcium (Ca^{2+}), magnesium (Mg^{2+}) and iron (Fe^{2+}) ions.

Sources of Poisoning

Oxalate poisoning in livestock generally occurs due to ingestion of oxalate producing plants. As many of these plants are palatable and form a large part of a ruminant's diet. Plants with more than 10 per cent of oxalic acid are considered as potentially dangerous upon feeding. Plant species which are of toxicological significance varies from country to country, but consumption of any plant rich in oxalate could be potentially toxic. Principal oxalate producing plants belong to the genus Rumex or genera of the family Chenopodiaceae and Oxalidaceae.

Plants Involved in Oxalate Poisoning

Scientific Name	Common Name	Active Ingredient
Amaranthus retroflexus	Red-root/Pig-weed amaranth, Spinach	Potassium acid oxalates
Spinacia oleracea		
Xanthosoma sagittifolium	Arrow leaf elephant ear	Calcium oxalates as raphides
Opuntia ficus - indica	Pricky pear	Soluble oxalates (sodium and potassium)

Scientific Name	Common Name	Active Ingredient
Beta vulgaris	Beet root, sugar beat	
Bassia hyssopifolia	Bassia	
Chenopodium album	Lamb's quarter, White goosefoot	
Halogeton glomeratus (34 per cent of soluble oxalates on DM basis)	Halogeton	Soluble oxalates
Sarcobatus vermiculatus (10-20 per cent of soluble oxalates on DM basis)	Greasewood	
Oxalis stricta	Sorrel	Potassium acid oxalates
Rumex crispus	Dock	Potassium acid oxalates
Rheum rhabarbarum	Rhubarb	Malonic acid and Potassium oxalates

Generally oxalate containing plants can be categorized into two groups: (1) Acid oxalate group ($HC_2O_4^-$) examples include Oxalis, Rumex species and (2) Oxalate ion ($C_2O_4^-$) group, occur in Halogeton, Sarcobatus, Amaranthus *etc.* Plants contain insoluble calcium oxalates as Raphides, which are sharp, needle shaped crystals containing gelantinous substance. Upon ingestion of these plants by animals, this gelatinous substance comes in contact with oral mucosa causing corrosive damage due to liberation of free oxalic acid.

Speceis Susceptibility

1. Ruminants are less susceptible, but prolonged grazing by cattle and sheep on tropical grasses causes severe hypocalcemia.
2. High levels of oxalates in beet tops resulted in hypocalcemia and hypomagnesmia in ewes.
3. In horses oxalates cause disturbance in bone minerals calcium and phosphorous by excessive mobilization. The demineralized bones become fibrotic and mishapen causing lameness and 'Big head'condition.

Factors Effecting Toxicity

Ruminants are more tolerant to oxalate poisoning than non-ruminants (horses), because rumen bacteria (*Oxalobacter formigenes*) can metabolise the oxalates into formic acid and carbondioxide. However, it is slow growing bacteria, hence in adapted cattle and sheep show gradually increase in tolerance to higher amounts of oxalates due to enhanced degradation activity by bacteria. Soluble oxalates such as sodium and potassium oxalates occurs rich in plant speceis such as *Agave, Beta, Bassia, Chenopodium, Halogeton, Oxalis, Rheum, Rumex, Sarcobatus* and *Setaria* genera and upon Consumption cause systemic toxicity. Soluble oxalate toxicity is species dependent, monogastric animals are more susceptible.

At neutral pH, plant oxalates occur as soluble form (oxalic acid, oxalate) or insoluble form (calcium oxalte). In monogastric animals when exposed to gastric pH (<2) even highly insoluble form becomes soluble. It is the soluble form causing more toxicity. Ruminants are less prone to chronic poisoning but are commonly poisoned when they are exposed to high oxalate concentrations in a short period of time, where there is no time for its body to adapt. Horses and monogastric animals are more susceptible to chronic poisoning when exposed to low oxalate for continuous period and less frequently to acute poisoning.

Toxicokinetics

Oxalaic acid is naturally produced in the body during metabolism of ascorbic acid, etheylene glycol, glyoxylic acid, glycolic acid and glycol. In case of Primary hyper oxaluria - which is classified into Primary hyper oxaluria type-I, deficiency of alanine:glyoxalate aminotransferase occur and in Primary hyper oxaluria type-II, defeceincy of glycolate reductase-hydroxy pyruvate reductase seen. In both conditions glyoxolate and glycolate failed to metabolise as glycolic acid leading to oxalate formation through alternate pathway.

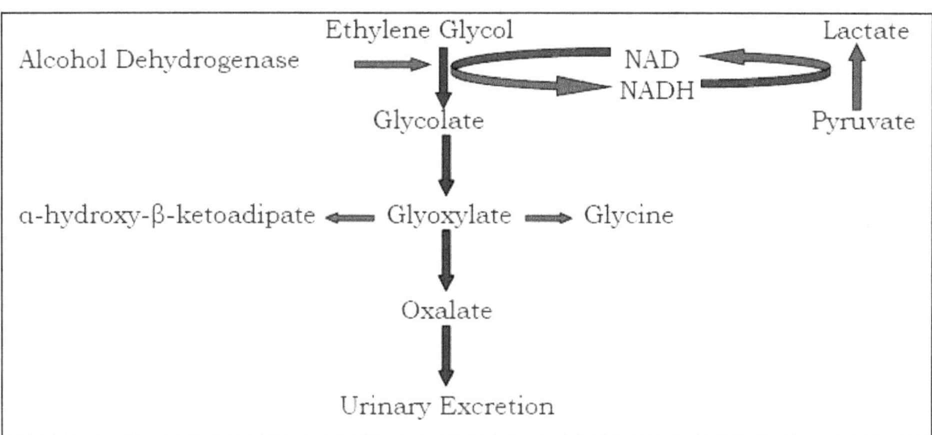

Figure 10.1: Oxalate Synthesis Pathway.

The amount of free oxalate available in the body depends on the levels of free calcium ions as they bind with oxalates in gut. In general, in ruminants, fate of oxalates may have four possible metabolic pathways upon consumption;

1. Degradation by rumen bacteria.
2. Consumption of soluble oxalates along with diet rich in calcium, they form insoluble calcium oxalate crystals in intestine and eliminated as such in faeces without being absoprbed into body.
3. When dietary calcium is low, these soluble oxalates get absorbed into blood stream from intestine, through blood vessels reach rumen

vasculature, cerebral vessels, filtered in to renal tubules where they bind with calcium to form insoluble calcium oxalate crystals.

4. Upon ingestion insoluble oxalate containing plants, these oxalates are eliminated as such through faeces, without being abosrbed into body.

Mechanism of Toxicity

In acute poisoning, the soluble oxalates are readily absorbed from the gastro-intestinal tract and clinical signs occur within 1-2 hours of post ingestion. In monogastric animals acidic pH favors the absorption of oxalic acid, whereas alkaline rumen pH enhances calcium oxalate formation, which gets precipitated decreasing potential systemic absorption. Absorbed soluble oxalates readily undergo glomerular filtration, but they are precipitated as calcium oxalate monohydrate (COM) crystal on renal tubules by binding with calcium.

It is reported that calcium oxalate monohydrate (COM) crystals, not oxalates are responsible for mitochondrial dysfunction, by altering its permeability transition. Chronic deposition of these crystals in renal tubules results in severe renal tubular necrosis called as oxalate nephrosis. Crystals may also occur on rumen vasculature where oxalate content is high and in few poisoning cases present in cerebral vessels, clinically associated with neurological signs.

Results of oxalate poisoning usually depends on location of crystals.

(i) If occur in GIT, causes irritation, which is seen as diaorrhea in sheep, upon secondary fungal infection cause hepatitis and rumenitis.

(ii) In blood causes hypocalcemia, by precipitating calcium as calcium oxalate. The decreased level of blood calcium is responsible for hypo motility of GI tract, which is commonly seen in oxalate poisoning.

(iii) Acute nephrosis and uremia is seen if calcium oxalate crystals precipitate in renal tubules. Oxalates form caliculi in kidneys, urethra, and bladder if consumed in small amounts for a prolonged period time.

(iv) In Australia, horses fed on *Setaria sphacelata* grass, which contains ammonium oxalate and also low in calcium caused osteodystropic fibrosa – metabolic bone disease.

Symptoms

Signs of toxicity usually occur within 2-6 hours of ingestion of toxic amount. Affected animals usually exhibit weakness, muscle tremors, staggering gait, rapid labored breathe, rapid pulse, diaorrhea is seen initially due to irritation followed by rumen atony due to hypocalemia, dilated pupils, haemorrhages, excessive salivation seen as froth at mouth, strain while urination due to calculi occur at urethra, urine may be red-brown. Coma and death of animal occurs within 10 hours of ingestion.

Diagnosis

By estimating the levels of serum calcium, they may drop to 20 per cent of normal condition at time of death. Albuminuria, haematuria, elevated BUN and creatinine levels. Analysis of suspected plant material by gas chromatography for quantification of oxalates is helpful to predict the risk associated and potential of poisoning. Calcium oxalate monohydrate binding protein (45-kd) is a promoter of calcium-oxalate kidney disease, which can be used as diagnostic marker for calcium-oxalate stones.

Differential Diagnosis

The condition should be differentiated from hypocalcaemia at parturition, lactation tetany, forced exercise, starvation.

Post-mortem Findings

Sigmoid flexure of bull and ram, urethral process of sheep will show the presence of calculi. Cystitis, urethritis, swollen kidney, cortex and medulla are separated by a grey line where oxalates accumulate. Histopathology of renal tubule contains small, rhomboid, transparent oxalate crystals. Crystals also occur in rumen wall. Hemorrhages are seen in GIT, cerebral blood vessels due to anticoagulant action.

Treatment

However toxicity associated with oxalates cannot be avoided but altered by using calcium supplements and antioxidant therapy. Supportive therapy includes IV or SC administration of calcium borogluconate 50-100ml in sheep and 500ml in cattle. Calcium supplement can not usually save the life of animal because during toxicity imbalance of other ions such as sodium and potassium during calcium precipitation. Flushing of kidney by force fed water; dextrose solution IV is also helpful.

Prevention

- ☆ Horses should not be fed on oxalate rich forages, as it causes nutritional disorders.
- ☆ Cattle and sheep should be gradually accustomed to oxalate rich diet, as it helps in enhanced activity of oxalate degrading rumen bacteria.
- ☆ Supplement diet with calcium rich sources as di-calcium phosphate, as dietary calcium can absorb oxalates from intestine, without being absorbed.
- ☆ Mixing of the diet with low oxalate containing plants, helps in reducing the overall intake of oxalte rich plants.
- ☆ Soaking the feed in water and later straining of the water, can also reduce oxalate content in the feed, decreases the toxicity.

Chapter 11

Mycotoxins

☆ *Rajeev Kumar, A.P. Suthar and C.V. Savalia*

A mycotoxin is derived from Greek word "myco", meaning mold and "toxin", a poison of biological origin. Several metabolites of mold and fungi have been identified as mycotoxin. The term mycotoxin was coined in 1962 in an unusual veterinary crisis near London, England, in which around 100,000 turkeys died. Mycotoxicosis is the term used to describe poisoning of a biological system by a mycotoxin. Mycotoxin is a toxic secondary metabolite produced by the fungus organism which is capable of causing disease as well as death in animals and humans. One mold species may produce different mycotoxins.

Because of their pharmacological activity, some mycotoxins or their derivatives have found use as drugs *e.g.*, antibiotics and growth promoters. Fungi are major plant pathogens but not a major disease causing agent in vertebrates. Animal exposure to mycotoxins may result from consumption of plant derived foods that are contaminated with toxins and the carryover them in animal products such as meat and eggs or exposure to air and dust containing toxins. The predisposing factors of mycotoxicosis are moisture, temperature, aeration, substrate availability and host stress. Currently, more than 300 mycotoxins are known, attention is focused mainly on those that have proven deterimental effects.

Classification

Classification of mycotoxins based on their target organs and systems.

Target Organ or System	Responsible Toxins
Liver	Aflatoxins, Rubratoxin, Sporodesmin, Penicillinic acid.
Kidney	Ochratoxins, Citrinin
Reproductive organ	Zearalenone, Zearalenol, T-2 Toxin
Nervous system	Fumonisins, Salframin, Citreoviridin, Patulin
Circulatory system	Ergot alkaloids

The principal classes of mycotoxins include a metabolite of *Aspergillus flavus* and *Aspergillus parasiticus*. In dairy cattle, problem arises from the transformation of Aflatoxin B_1 (AFB_1) and Aflatoxin B_1 (AFB_2) into hydroxylated metabolites Aflatoxin M_1 (AFM_1) and Aflatoxin M_2 (AFM_2), respectively. These are found in milk and milk products obtained from livestock if animals have ingested contaminated feed. AFB_1 is most potent hepatocarcinogenic substance, which has been proven to also be genotoxic, also.

1. Aflatoxin

Aflatoxins are the toxic metabolites of the saprotrophic and pathogenic fungus of *Aspergillus flavus* and *Aspergillus parasiticus*. They grow rapidly and generate toxic in grains and feed stored under aerobic conditions with moisture more than 15 per cent and 24-25°C temperature. Peanuts, cottonseed meal and cake are affected frequently. Although 13 aflatoxins have been identified; aflatoxin B_1, B_2, G_1 and G_2 are the major types. This grouping has been done according to their fluorescence characteristics. B_1 and B_2 produce blue while G_1 and G_2 produce green fluorescence. The AFB_1 metabolite is important because of toxicity and concentration in moldy feeds. The order of toxicity is $B_1 > G_1 > B_2 > G_2$. Metabolites of B_1 and B_2 are excreted in milk and are termed as M_1 and M_2. Aflatoxin B_1 is the most potent natural carcinogen.

Aflatoxins are polycyclic unsaturated compounds relatively heat resistant and not soluble in water. They are extractable in organic solvents and are unstable when expose to UV radiation. Addition of fungicidal drugs can prevent the growth of the mold, but will not destroy already developed mycotoxin. Ammoniation is helpful, but is not an approved procedure.

Toxicity

Milk products serve as an indirect source of aflatoxin. Aflatoxin is associated with both toxicity and carcinogenicity in animal and human populations. Death may occur in acute aflatoxicosis, whereas cancer, immune suppression, and "slow" pathological conditions in low dose exposure. The liver is the primary target organ. AFB_1 is potent carcinogen, mutagen and teratogen and liver damaging agent. Liver tumor is more common toxic effect.

Most susceptible animals include rabbit, duckling, mink, trout, dog, turkey and small pig. Animals like monkeys, WLH chick, rat, mice and hamster are quite resistant. Apart from age, sex, breed and strain of animal, other important factors include riboflavin, exposure to light, diet low in protein, cholin and vitamin B_{12}. Animals on protein, vitamin E and selenium deficient diet are more susceptible.

Mechanism of Action

AFB_1 binds to nuclear DNA and decreases synthesis of RNA ultimately reduces enzymes and protein. AFB_1 also combies to endoplasmic steroidal binding sites causing ribosomal disaggregation.

Clinical Symptoms

Acute symptoms include anorexia, depression, dyspnoea, coughing, nasal discharge, anemia, epistaxis, bloody faeces, convulsions and rapid death. Animals may develop jaundice, hypoprothrombinaemia, haematoma and haemorrhagic enteritis.

In chronic toxicity there is gradual decrease in feed efficiency, productivity and weight gain as well as rough hair coat, anaemia, enlarged abdomen, mild jaundice together with depression and anorexia. Abortion may also be noticed during pregnancy.

Post-mortem Lesions

Icterus, widespread petechial haemorrhages, haemorrhagic gastoenterisits, hepatic necrosis, enlarged liver, hepatic fibrosis, cirrhosis, ascitis, hydrothorax and oedema of the wall of the gall bladder.

Diagnosis

Diagnosis is made by estimation of serum liver enzymes. All the serum liver enzymes are elevated. Serum albumin and albumin:globulin ratio is decreased. Biochemical changes are secondary to cytotoxic actions of aflatoxins, include increased SGOT, SGPT and alkaline phosphatase, isocitric dehydrogenase and bilirubin. There is decrease in serum protein, NPN and urea. Synthesis of clotting proteins is also inhibited.

Aflatoxin levels can also be estimated using TLC (Thin-Layer Chromatography), GC (Gas Chromatography). Aflatoxin-M can be detected in milk and urine as bright greenish yellow florescence under UV light.

Treatment

Contaminated feed must be removed. Feed low in fat and high in protein must be fed. Activated charcoal, anabolic steroid stanazolol and oxyteracycline are useful. Hydrated sodium calcium aluminosilicate has a high affinity for aflatoxins and can adsorb aflatoxins. Use of vitamin E and selenium has been found to be useful in ameliorating the effects of aflatoxin. Use of Vitamin-B_{12} and vitamin-K are also useful.

2. Rubratoxin

Rubratoxins are produced by soil fungi *Penicillium rubrum* and *Penicillium purpurogenum*. Exposure to the toxin is through cereal grains, primarily corn. The rubratoxins occur in two forms *i.e.* rubratoxins A and B, with an unusual polycyclic structure containing stable anhydride functions. Toxicity is due to the presence of an α, β-unsaturated lactose ring in their structure. Rubratoxin-B is most toxic rubratoxin, which is hepatotoxic, mutagenic and teratogenic.

Male and female rats are equally susceptible. Rubratoxins are poorly soluble in water, insoluble in oils, and soluble in alcohol and esters. The toxins are stable at room temperature, but heating at 85-100°C for two hours may destroy rubratoxins in feeds. Most of the toxin is excreted in urine as parent compound in rats and slightly excreted in feces.

Produce mutagenic, embryocidal, teratogenic toxicity in mice. Clinical syndrome is similar to acute aflatoxicosis. Post mortem lesions characterized by hepatotoxicity, nephrosis and general bleeding tendency. Congestion and hemorrhage in liver, kidney and spleen. Early midzonal hepatic necrosis is observed.

3. Fumonisin

Fumonisins are mycotoxins produced by the fungus *Fusarium moniliforme* primarily in corn. Several climatic factors predispose to fungal growth and toxin production such as: midsummer drought, an early wet fall, fluctuating warm and cold temperatures, accompanied by an early frost and delayed harvests. Horses, ponies, and donkeys may develop leukoencephalomalacia and liver failure. Other species like as swine develops pulmonary edema and rabbits may develop renal failure in rabbits.

Fumonisins (B_1 and B_2) are cancer promoting metabolites of *Fusarium proliferatum* and *Fusarium verticillioides* that have a long-chain hydrocarbon unit which plays a role in their toxicity. Fumonisin B_1 (FB_1) is most toxic. It causes leukoencephalomalacia in equine and pulmonary edema in porcine and promote tumor in rats. FB_1 is the diester of propane-1, 2, 3-tricarboxylic acid and a pentahydroxyeicosane in which the C11 and C15 hydroxy groups are esterified with the terminal carboxy group of propane-1, 2, 3-tricarboxylic acid. Fumonisins are soluble in methanol and stable in acetonitrile-water (1:1) at 25°C, stable in buffer solutions over the pH range 4.8-9 at 78 °C.

Mechanisms of Action

FB_1 apparently causes toxic effects by inhibiting the action of sphingosine N-acyltransferase, an enzyme involved in the conversion of sphinganine and sphingosine into sphingolipids. Inhibition of N-acyltransferase causes, increase in sphinganine concentration in tissues. Sphingolipids are important in regulation of cell growth, differentiation, and neoplastic transformation. Alteration in sphingolipid concentrations and functions especially in the vasculature contribute fumonisin toxicosis.

In swine, fumonisin causes damage to hepatocyte membranes causing release of membrane fragments to circulation. These are trapped in the lung where they alter capillary permeability resulting in pulmonary edema. Cardiac failure and pulmonary hypertension due to pulmonary vasoconstriction may occur in swine.

Clinical Symptoms

(a) Neurotoxic Syndrome

This syndrome is termed as equine leukoencephalomalacia (ELEM); although earlier nomenclatures include blind staggers, cerebritis, leukoencephalitis, encephalomyelitis, cornstalk disease, moldy corn poisoning, foraging disease, and cerebrospinal meningitis.

The clinical course is generally short. Death occurs within 2-3 days. Partial anorexia often observed early in the course. Anorexia coincides with paralysis of glossopharyngeal, lips and tongue, and subsequently loss the ability to grasp and chew food. Depression, ataxia, blindness, and hysteria are common. Head is often held low, especially when left alone. Incoordination, aimless walking, circling movement, and ataxia often occur. Head pressing, stupor and hyperesthesia are common. Hyperexcitability, profuse sweating, delirium, mania and convulsions are often present, especially terminally. Death may occur even without showing any previous signs.

(b) Hepatotoxic Syndrome

In horse usually icterus with hepatic degeneration is prominent. Oral petechial, edema of the face and submandibular space may also seen. Elevated bilirubin, liver enzymes are noticed. Terminal diaphoresis, coma, and sometimes clonic convulsions may be noted, presumably due to hepatoencephalopathy. Swine exhibit decline in feed consumption is usually the first sign.

If more toxin ingested, acute pulmonary edema and, often, death follows. At low doses, slowly progressive liver disease occurs. Poor performance, feed refusal, diarrhoea, weakness, and high mortality noticed in poultry. Rats exhibit hepatic neoplasia while rabbits show sudden renal failure. In human, oesophageal cancer is suspected to be related to consumption of fumonisin contaminated corn.

Diagnosis

Diagnosis is based on clinical signs and lesions. Characteristic liquefactive necrosis of white matter in the brain may be only histologically evident even in lethally affected horses.

Treatment

Isolate affected horses to prevent other horses from traumatizing them or vice versa. Thiamine may be useful. Activated charcoal and a saline cathartic for the first two days could be tried. Corn in diet should be avoided. Maintenance of hydration and other supportive therapy have been found to be useful.

4. Citreoviridin

Citreoviridin is a neurotoxic mycotoxin from *Penicillium spp.*, *Aspergillus terreus*, and several other related fungi. Citreoviridin is soluble in benzene, ethanol, chloroform, ether, dichloromethane. Citreoviridin is hardly soluble in water and hexane. It can cause ascending paralysis with convulsions and respiratory paralysis resulting in respiratory arrest. Cardiovascular and respiratory failure may occur within three days after the initial onset of paralysis.

5. Patulin

Patulin is a mycotoxin produced by *Penicilium* spp. and *Aspergillus* spp. It is an inhibitor of RNA polymerase. It is produced in apples, pears, grapes, barley, malt, rice, and wheat straw. Cattle consuming contaminated feed have reportedly exhibited an ascending paralysis of motor nerves with convulsions, excitement and cerebral hemorrhage. Lesions may include pulmonary and cerebral edema, ascites, and congestion of liver, spleen, and kidneys.

Patulin is a heat stable polyketide lactone, soluble in low pH water and organic solvents. It is not destroyed by pasteurization or thermal denaturation. However, stability following fermentation is lessened. It is reactive with sulfur dioxide, so antioxidant and antimicrobial agents may be useful to destroy it.

6. Ochratoxin

Ochratoxin-A (OTA) is produced by *Aspergillus ochraceus*, *Aspergillus carbonarius*, *Aspergillus melleus*, *Aspergillus sclerotiorum*, *Aspergillus sulphureus* and *Pichia verrucossum*. OTA is most common of all the ochratoxin and has the greatest toxicological significance. Ochratoxins represent 9 isocoumarin compounds synthesized from phenylalanine. OTA consists of a polyketide-derived dihydroiso-coumarin moiety linked through the 12-carboxy group to phenylalanine. The optimum temperature range for toxin production is 12°C-25°C. It is a colourless crystalline compound, exhibiting blue fluorescence under UV light.

OTA is frequent natural contaminant of many foodstuffs *viz.*, as cocoa beans, coffee beans, cassava flour, cereals, fish, peanuts, dried fruits, wine, poultry eggs and milk. The toxin occurs in barley, sorghum wheat, corn, dried beans, rye, oats, mixed feeds, and peanuts. Toxicity has been demonstrated in swine, ducklings, chickens, turkeys, and dogs.

7. Trichothecene

The trichothecene (TCT) mycotoxins comprise a vast group of fungal metabolites with the same basic structure. Several fungal genera are capable of producing TCT; however, most of them have been isolated from *Fusarium spp.* All TCT contain an epoxide at C-12 and C-13 positions, which is responsible for their toxicological activity. At the cellular level, the main toxic effect of TCT mycotoxins appears to be a primary inhibition of protein synthesis. TCT affect actively dividing cells such as those lining the gastrointestinal tract, the skin, lymphoid and erythroid cells. Type-A and type-B are commonly occur natural toxins. Types-A and B trichothecene are distinguished by the presence or absence of a carbonyl group at the C-8 position.

Trichothecenes belong to a class of sesquiterpene lactones known as 12, 13-epoxy- trichothecenes. On the basis of their molecular structure, trichothecenes are divided into two group: the macrocyclic (*e.g.* satratoxin, verrucarin and roridin) and the non-microcyclic (*e.g.*T-2, diacetoxyscirpenol and deoxynivalenol) trichothecenes. But known and of greatest concern are non-microcyclic trichothecenes and out of all trichothecenes T-2 is most cytotoxic. Trichothecenes are poorly soluble in water, but are soluble in organic solvents and fats. These toxins resist chemical and environmental decomposition and persist in field indefinitely.

The toxic action of TCT results in extensive necrosis of the oral mucosa and skin in contact with the toxin, acute effect on the digestive tract and impairment of bone marrow and immune function. Toxin production is more in high humidity and temperatures of 6–24°C. Trichothecenes have been detected in corn, wheat, barley, oats, rice, rye, vegetables, and other crops. They are common contaminants of poultry feeds and feedstuffs and their adverse effects on poultry health and productivity have been studied extensively.

8. Zearalenone

Zearalenone is a mycotoxin produced by *Fusarium graminearum*. It is a non-steroidal compound that exhibits oestrogen like activity in farm animals like cattle, sheep and pigs. Zearalenone is a phenolic resorcyclic acid lactone with potent oestrogenic properties.

Zearalenone is 6-(10-hydroxy-6-oxo-trans-1-undecanyl) β-resorcylic-acid-lactone. Zearalenone is soluble in alkaline solutions, ether, benzene, acetonitrile, methyl chloride, chloroform, acetone and alcohols, but insoluble in water. It is heat stable, which makes it difficult to remove. It is not destroyed by addition of propionic acid or mould retardants.

Mechanisms of Action

The toxin is absorbed readily from the gastrointestinal tract and excreted in faeces, urine and milk. Enterohepatic recycling increases duration of action. Bind to cytosolic receptors for oestradiol 17β. This complex binds to oestradiol site on DNA and inhibits specific RNA synthesis. Functions as weak oestrogen and inhibits follicle stimulating hormone. This in turn inhibits preovulatory ovarian follicle maturation.

Clinical Symptoms

Swine are more susceptible. In cattle, causes infertility. Hypoestrogenism is noticed in prepubertal females. Other signs include are nymphomania, anoestrus, vaginitis and mammary enlargement in heifers.

Treatment

Treatment with activated charcoal, supportive therapy and prostaglandins is useful.

9. Moniliformin

Moniliformin is produced by several Fusarium species (mainly *Fusarium proliferatum*) and is usually found on the corn kernel. It can be transferred to next generation crops and survive for years in the soil. Although both AFB_1 and moniliformin are produced by the same fungal species (*F. proliferatum*), no structural resemblance is found between the two toxins. Moniliformin is an ionic compound forming sodium and potassium salts and is soluble in water and polar solvents.

10. Ergon Alkaloid

The most prominent member of this group is *Claviceps purpurea* ("rye ergot fungus"). Which grows on rye and related plants, and produces alkaloids that causes ergotism in humans and other mammals who consume contaminated grains. *Claviceps purpurea* has three varieties, which differ in their host specificity: G_1 - land grasses of open meadows and fields; G_2 - grasses from moist, forest, and mountain habitats; G_3 - salt marsh grasses (*Spartina, Distichlis*). Ergot alkaloids are derivatives of lysergic acid. The important ergot alkaloids are ergotamine, ergometrine, ergocryptine, ergocornine, ergocristine and ergosine. The collective extract of ergot is called ergotoxin. Chemically, ergot alkaloids fall into two major categories *viz.*, compounds with an amine side-chain include ergometrine and those with an amino acid side chain include ergotamine.

The ergot alkaloids are among the most fascinating fungal metabolites. They are classified as indole alkaloids and are derived from a tetracyclic ergoline ring system. They are produced as a toxic cocktail of alkaloids in the sclerotia of species of *Claviceps*, which are common pathogens of various grass species.

Ergotism is still an important problem in animals. The principal animals at risk are cattle, sheep, pig, and chicken. Nowadays it is very rare, because the normal grain cleaning and milling processes remove most of the ergot. In addition, the alkaloids that are the causative agents of ergotism are relatively unstable usually destroyed during baking and cooking.

Clinical symptoms of ergotism in animals include gangrene, abortion, convulsions, suppression of lactation and hypersensitivity.

Pure ergotamine has been used for the treatment of migraine headaches in humans. Other ergot derivatives are used as prolactin inhibitors, in the treatment of parkinsonism, and in cases of cerebrovascular insufficiency. The therapeutic administration of ergot alkaloids poses sporadic cases of human ergotism.

Food and Feed Additives

☆ *Rajeev Ranjan and Pavan Kumar*

Food additives are substances which have little or no nutritive value, but are used to improve the foods or animal feed in many different ways such as providing better consistency, aroma, texture, color, nutrition, flavor and storage or shelf life. Some additives have been used for the prolonging of the life. In the second half of the 20th century, large numbers of additives have been introduced that is both natural and artificial origin. These substances are added to food products during the processing, storage, and packaging. *e.g.*, antimicrobials, anabolic steroid and hormone, non-protein nitrogen (NPN), common salt (Sodium chloride), anticaking agents, coloring agent, flavor enhancer, antioxidants, non-nutritive or non-sugar sweeteners, preservative, stabilizers, thickeners, bulking agents, *etc.*

Purpose to Use Food Additives

Food additives serve four major purposes in our foods-

1. To provide nutrition
2. To maintain product quality and freshness
3. To aid in the processing and preparation of foods
4. To make foods appealing

To Provide Nutrition

It improves or maintains the nutritional quality of food. For example-

☆ The addition of iodine to salt has contributed to the virtual elimination of simple goiter.

☆ The addition of vitamin-D to milk and other dairy products has accomplished the same thing with respect to rickets.

☆ Niacin in bread, corn meal and cereals has helped eliminate pellagra, a disease characterized by central nervous system and skin disorders.

☆ Thiamine and iron are used for further fortification in the diet.

To Maintain Product Quality and Freshness

Fresh foods do not stay for long periods of time. They rapidly deteriorate, turn rancid and spoil. Food additives delay significantly this deterioration and prevent spoilage caused by growth of microorganisms, bacteria and yeast and also by oxidation or oxygen in air coming into contact with the foods. For example-

☆ Cut slices of fresh fruits rapidly turn brown due to this oxidation process. However, placing these slices in juice from lemons, limes or oranges can stop this process. Food processors do the same thing by using ascorbic acid (the principal active ingredient in citrus juice).

☆ Propionates, which naturally occur in cheese, are used similarly in bakery goods to prevent the growth of molds and to improve or maintain the nutritional quality of food.

To Aid in the Processing and Preparation of Foods

Additives maintain certain desirable qualities associated with various foods. For example:

☆ Emulsifiers such as lecithin from soybeans maintain mixture and improve texture in dressings and other foods. They are used in ice cream where smoothness is desired, in breads to increase volume and impart fine grain quality, and in cake mixes to achieve better consistency.

☆ Pectin, derived from citrus peels and used in jellies and preserves when thickening is desired, belongs in the category of stabilizers and thickeners.

☆ Leaveners used to make breads and biscuits, include yeast, baking powder and baking soda.

☆ Humectants, like sorbitol that naturally occurs in apples, are used when moisture retention is necessary, such as in the packaging of shredded coconut.

To Make Foods Appealing

The majority of food additives are most often used for this purpose. Unless foods look appetizing and appeal to our senses, they will most likely go uneaten and valuable nutrients will be lost.

☆ Food additives such as sweeteners, flavor enhancers, and coloring agents are included by food processors because we demand foods that look good and taste.

Classification of Food Additives

Food additives can be divided into several groups based on their use or function.

(i) Anticaking agents

(ii) Coloring agent

(iii) Color retention agent

(iv) Flavor enhancer or flavoring agents

(v) Antioxidants

(vi) Non-nutritive or non-sugar sweeteners

(vii) Preservative

(viii) Stabilizers

(ix) Thickeners

(x) Anti foaming agents

(x) Humectants

(xi) Bulking agents

(xii) Glazing agents

(i) Anticaking Agents

Anticaking agents are added to finely powdered or crystalline food to prevent the formation of lumps (caking) or sticking and for easing packaging, transport and consumption. Sodium aluminosilicate or sodium silicoaluminate is present in many commercial table salts as well as dried milk, sugar products, and flours as recommended concentrations in food additive. *e.g.* sodium aluminosilicate, calcium silicate, dimethyl polysiloxane, *etc.*

(ii) Coloring Agents

Color additive or agents are any dye, pigment or substance that added to food to make the food more attractive and to replace the color lost during preparation. *e.g.*, amaranth and tartrazine.

Amaranth is an azodye and its trisodium salts are used as coloring agents. The FAO/WHO recommended its acceptable daily intake as 0-1.5 mg/kg. It produces malignant tumors in rats and may produced liver damage including vacuolization and fatty degeneration. For this reason, FDA and several countries have banned the use of amaranth in food, drugs and cosmetics.

Tartrazine is a coal tar derivative azodye and large number of food product like soft drink, noodles, pickels, chips, jam, jelly, ice cream, candy, sauces, biscuits *etc.* contain this agent. It is known to be least toxic coloring agents. The acute oral LD_{50} of tartrazine is 12-17 mg/kg body weight in mice. FDA has set its daily intake at 0-7.5 mg/kg. Anaphylactic shock with common symptoms of urticaria, asthma and purpura has reported in sensitive human.

(iii) Color Retention Agent

These agents are used to hold the existing natural color or protect the food from losing its inherent color. Many of these agents work by absorbing or binding to oxygen before it can damage the foods. It is added to wines, fruit and vegetable based drinks, juices, baby foods and fat containing cereal based foods, such as biscuits. *e.g.*, ascorbic acid.

(iv) Flavoring and Flavor Enhancer

Flavoring agent may be derived from natural or artificially origin that give food a particular taste or smell and improve the acceptability of food. Flavor enhancers or agents used to enhance existing flavor of food. Monosodium glutamate is most common flavor enhancer extracted from natural source, whereas safrole, maltol and methyl anthranilate derived artificially.

Methyl anthranilate is a colorless liquid which has sweet grape like flavor. It is found in the essential oils of orange, lemon and jasmine and has been used by the food and drug industry. Its oral LD_{50} in rats and mice has been calculated to be 3900 and 2910 mg/kg body weight, respectively. Allergic reactions produced by methyl anthranilate on human skin, so it is being prohibited for use in cosmetic industry.

Safrole is typically extracted from root bark or fruit of sassafras plants in the form of sassafras oil. Safrole has a characteristic candy-shop aroma and was once widely used as a food additive. The food and drug administration (FDA) has barred its use, due to its mild carcinogenic properties.

(v) Antioxidants

Oxidative deterioration produces undesirable change in color, flavor, nutritive value and sometime other toxic materials in food. These agents retard the deterioration, rancidity and discoloration due to oxidation. Carotenes as well as vitamin-C and E used as antioxidant and act as preservatives by inhibiting the effects of oxygen on food. They extend the shelf life of the food, if used properly.

Ascorbic acid act as a coenzyme in some enzymatic reaction and used as antioxidant that protects against oxidative stress. It is safe in recommended concentration but ingestion of relatively large dose may cause indigestion, nervous symptoms and urinary oxalate stone. World health organization (WHO) has recommended its daily intake should be less than 0.25 mg/kg body weight.

(vi) Non-Nutritive Sweetener

Non nutritive sweeteners (also called as sugar substitutes or artificial non-sugar sweeteners) are substances that are used instead of sugars to sweeten foods, beverages and certain medications. These are compounds with many times the sweetness of sucrose. So they are required in much less quantity and energy contribution is often negligible. Some sugar substitutes are natural and some are synthetic. These include saccharin, sodium cyclamate, aspartame, sucralose, neotame and acesulfame potassium.

Saccharin is one of the most commonly used artificial sweeteners. It is about 300 to 500 times as sweet as sugar (sucrose) and is often used to improve the taste of toothpastes, dietary foods, and dietary beverages. The bitter aftertaste of saccharin is often minimized by blending it with other sweeteners. In the body it does not affect insulin levels and has effectively no food energy. It is used as sodium or calcium salt. The oral LD_{50} of sodium saccharin in mice and rat is 17.5 and 14.2

gm/kg body weight, respectively. Sodium saccharin induces bladder tumor in male rats when administered at high level for longer time.

Aspartame is a non carbohydrate sweetener and derived from the two amino acids aspartic acid and phenylalanine. It is about 200 times as sweet as sugar and can be used as a tabletop sweetener, gelatins, beverages, and chewing gum. When cooked or stored at high temperatures or high pH, aspartame breaks down into its constituent amino acids. This makes aspartame undesirable as a baking sweetener. It does not have a bitter aftertaste like saccharin, it may not taste exactly like sugar. When eaten, aspartame is metabolized into its original amino acids. Because it is so intensely sweet, relatively little of it is needed to sweeten a food product, and is thus useful for reducing the number of calories in a product. Some studies have indicated that aspartame induces cancer as well as neurological or psychiatric side effects.

(vii) **Preservative**

Preservatives are agents which prevent or inhibit spoilage of food due to bacteria, fungi and other microorganisms. Use of antibiotics as preservatives may lead to danger of developing resistant strain of pathogens. Some synthetic compounds are available which are widely used as food preservatives. *e.g.*, benzoic acid and sorbic acid.

Benzoic acid and its sodium salt (sodium benzoate) is extensively used as food preservative and inhibits the microbial growth of by lowering the intracellular pH to 5 or less. The used of benzoic acid ranges from 0.05 to 0.1 per cent. The acute oral LD_{50} of sodium benzoate in rats, rabbits and dogs is 2700, 2000 and 2000 mg/kg body weight, respectively. Large doses of benzoic acid may cause abdominal pain, sore throat, nausea, vomition, hypersensitivity, enlargement of liver and kidney.

Sorbic acid and its salt (sodium sorbate, potassium sorbate and calcium sorbate) are used as preservatives in food and drinks. The salts of sorbic acid are preferred over the acid because more water solubility. The oral LD_{50} in rats is more than 10.5 gm/kg body weight. Ingestion of large dose may produce gastrointestinal disturbance.

(viii) **Stabilizers**

Stabilizer is an additive to food which helps to preserve its structure or give foods a firmer texture. They help to stabilize emulsion and improve consistency. Some hydrocolloids like agar, gelatin, pectin, alginate, cellulose, *etc.*, are frequently used as stabilizer.

(ix) **Thickeners**

Thickeners are substances which, when added to the mixture, increase its viscosity without substantially modifying its other properties. Edible thickeners are commonly used to thicken sauces and soup without altering their taste. Important member of the thickener are protein (collagen, egg whites and gelatin), starches (arrowroot, potato starch, corn starch and tapioca) and vegetable gums (alginin, guar gum and xanthan gum).

(x) Anti-foaming Agents

Antifoaming agents are additive that prevent formation of foam or added to break foam already formed in foods. The essential feature of this agent is a low viscosity and a facility to spread rapidly on foaming surface. Antifoaming agents are included in variety of foods such as chicken nuggets in the form of polydimethoxysiloxane. Silicon oil is also added to cooking oil to prevent foaming in deep frying. Some antifoaming agents like simethicone which is an active ingredient in drug to relieve bloat.

(xi) Humectants

These are agents which prevent foods from drying out or retain moisture and maintain the moisture content of the food. Both honey and glucose syrup is commonly used as humectants for their water absorption and sweet flavor properties. Some food humectants like sucrose, glycerol and its triester (triacetin) are used for the purpose of controlling viscosity and texture.

(xii) Bulking Agents

Bulking agent is a food additive that increases food volume or weight of food without affecting its nutritive value. Bulking agents are widely used in low calorie foods, meal replacements, pastries and most processed foods. These agents can be used as weight loss aid for their ability of delivering fullness and decreased appetite. Some common bulking agents are psyllium husk, methyl cellulose and pectin.

(xiii) Glazing Agents

Glazing agents provide a waxy or shiny appearance and provide protective coating to foods. e.g. stearic acid, lanolin, paraffin, beeswax, etc.

Feed Additives

Feed additives are pharmacological or nutritional substances used in animal nutrition for the various purposes either for improving the quality of feed or growth and performance enhancers or to control infectious disease. It is used in small quantity, but improper use may cause poisoning in the subject animals or undesirable residues in food for human consumption produced by the animals. The use of additives is strictly controlled by legislation in most countries.

Antimicrobials

Antimicrobials and other drugs are used by veterinarians and livestock owners to increase the size of livestock, poultry, and other farmed animals. Antibiotics not only use for the treatment or prophylaxis of infection but at sub therapeutic doses in animal feed, it promote growth and improve feed efficiency in animals. The use of some drugs is banned in some countries due to food contamination or concern about increasing antibiotic resistance.

Certain antibiotics, when given in low or sub therapeutic doses, it improve the feed conversion efficiency (more output, such as muscle or milk, for a given amount of feed) and/or may promote greater growth, most likely by affecting gut flora. The indiscriminate use of antibiotics as a growth promoter may be problematic for future. Sub therapeutic use of antibiotics results in increase bacterial resistance. Some important class of antibiotics is being used commonly are as follows:

Antibiotic Used as Growth Promoters in Livestock Production

Drugs	*Effects*
Virginiamycin	: Promotes growth
Tylosin	: Increase weight gain
Lasalocid	: Increase feed conversion ratio
Bambermycin	: Increase feed conversion ratio and promotes growth
Monensin	: Increase feed conversion ratio and increase weight gain
Salinomycin	: Increase feed conversion ratio and increase weight gain

Anabolic Steroid and Hormone

The U. S. Food and Drug Administration (FDA) have approved a number of steroid hormone drugs for use in beef cattle and sheep, including natural estrogen, progesterone, testosterone, and their synthetic versions. These drugs increase the animal's growth rate, the efficiency by which they convert the feed into meat, and the leanness of their meat.

Some supplemental hormones (gonadotropins, progestogens and estrogens) can be given to dairy cows to extend milk production. These are also useful to synchronize estrus during the breeding season, increase the ovulation rate and incidence of multiple births, induce fertile mating during anestrous and induce early puberty.

Excess or long term supplementation of the anabolic steroids, delays puberty, premature epiphyseal fusion, stunted growth, impair udder development and increase the incidence of dystokia in animals. Beside these effects in animals, human health is also adversely affected due to carcinogenic potential of residues of certain synthetic hormone in meat and milk.

Non-protein Nitrogen (NPN)

Non protein nitrogen is collection of some components such as urea, biurate, ammonium salt, which are not proteins but can be converted into proteins by microbes in ruminant stomach. Due to their lower cost compared to plant and animal proteins their inclusion in a diet can result in economic gain. Normal feeding rate for NPN products is 3 per cent of the grain ration or 1 per cent of the total ration.

When animal ingests large quantity of NPN mixed ration or accidentally ingest excess amount of ammoniated fertilizers cause a depression in growth and ammonia toxicity because microbes convert NPN to ammonia first before using that to make protein. Early signs in various species may include frothy salivation, grinding of teeth, muscles tremors, polyurea, ruminal atony, bellowing, and kicking at abdomen due to colic.

Common Salt (Sodium Chloride)

Sodium chloride is added to feed or ration to improve palatability and nutritional value. It play important role in nerve conduction, muscle contraction, correct osmotic balance and absorption of other nutrients. Sodium chloride may become toxic, when animal ingests excessive quantities salt and intake of water is limited. Sign of the salt poisoning are increased thrist, pruritis, salivation, vomition, urinary inconsistence or polyurea later anuria, diarrhea, and may cause constipation. Nervous sign include hyperthesia, partial or complete blindness or deafness, shivering or twitching and seizures.

Index